LIVE LONGER, LIVE BETTER: YOUR GUIDE TO LONGEVITY

UNLOCK THE SCIENCE OF AGING, MASTER PRACTICAL STRATEGIES, AND MAXIMIZE YOUR HEALTH AND HAPPINESS FOR A VIBRANT LIFE IN YOUR GOLDEN YEARS

KOOROSH NAGHSHINEH

CONTENTS

MEDICAL DISCLAIMER

This book is not meant to replace medical treatment.

.

HOW THIS BOOK CAME ABOUT

I come from a family whose members are generally blessed with a long life. Except in a few cases of cancer or accidental death, most of my grandparents, aunts, and uncles have lived (or continue to live) into their eighties and even a few well into their nineties. I have one uncle who is now one hundred years old.

This seems to be a blessing to most until you look closely at each of these people and find out how happy they really are in their old age. Some have a productive life until their last days. These seem to be generally happy and healthier than most.

Others fall into the pattern of complaining about living too long. They say things like: "All my friends are dead," "Why did God make me live this long and see my brothers and sisters pass away before me," "I am too old and suffering all these ailments," etc.

I have admired those of my relatives who lived a long time and seemed productive and generally happy and satisfied with their lives. I asked myself, "How can I be more like these people?" My search for answers brought me to the topic of longevity and the research that ended up in this book. I hope what I have learned and summarized in this book can also benefit you.

My hope and wish are that if I am blessed to live a long life, I can be more like those who make the best out of the time they are given. Be a productive member of society to my last days, keep learning, stay as healthy as possible, and continue to do some good in this world. I have heard the phrase "die with my boots on." That's what I imagine for myself.

FREE GIFTS FOR THE READER

Thank you for reading *Live Longer, Live Better: Your Guide to Longevity*. I hope you will find it insightful, inspiring, and, most importantly, practical. I hope it helps you live longer, happier, and healthier.

To help you get the best results as fast as possible, I have included the following additional bonus materials at no extra cost to you. These are:

- Longevity quiz
- Assessment of longevity factors
- Access to a weekly meal planner template
- Healthy recipes
- Exercises for improving your balance and health, including videos

To get your bonuses, please scan this image using your cell-phone camera.

Alternatively, you can go to this link:

https://www.betterbalanceforall.com

In both cases, you will be directed to the same website where you will create an account and receive access to this material. My goal is to continue to add useful material to this website to help you succeed in improving your health and life balance.

INTRODUCTION

"The various features and aspects of human life, such as longevity, good health, success, happiness, and so forth, which we consider desirable, are all dependent on kindness and a good heart." ~ Dalai Lama

Life has many stages. In our youth, we are builders and creators of our life. We try to figure out what we want to do and experiment with life until we settle on something. I am talking about a family, a career, a home, etc. All of these are our creations, whether we acknowledge that we are the person who created that we are the person who created 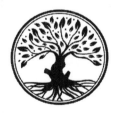 them or not. Then, at some point, usually, by our early forties, we find that we have hit our stride. We have a clear sense of our place in the world, our direction, our relationships, and our purpose.

But change is inevitable. Unexpected changes can knock us off our feet. For me, it was a divorce in my early forties and, years later, an unexpected retirement from my lengthy academic career. These are major life events. At each point of my journey, I've gone through significant changes that have deeply impacted me. I've had to reassess who I am, where I fit in the world and what my life means.

The way life changes forever differs for everyone.

Most people are afraid of change. We simply don't want to lose our point of comfort, especially if it is painful. We have gotten used to life the way it is. What are you used to? Do you fear change? What changes keep you awake at night? Declining health? Curtailing expenses? Early retirement? The kids leaving home? Divorce? Death of a loved one? These are only a few of the many reasons causing people like myself to experience increased anxiety, stress, and even fear over time. Sometimes aging can be scary because of the unexpected changes that accompany it.

Can you identify with this situation?

At a certain age, we all face the fact that we have fewer years left ahead of us than those we have already lived. Have you become aware of your mortality? Do you feel that you need to enjoy the time you have and live better than ever before? Then read on. This is what I found in my own journey as I looked for answers to these questions.

The Midlife Crisis

We all enter midlife between the ages of 40 and 60. This is an age often linked to a state of transformation. A time widely associated with changes in our life situation, possibly our health and wellness, fitness, and mental clarity.

Do you feel the pain and discomfort I am sharing here? The only reason why I can describe this state with so much accuracy is that I've experienced it firsthand. I've seen my friends go through similar battles, unsure how it will end. Or when. It is a time of uncertainty about where life is heading and our place in the future.

I think the greatest uncertainty for me was wondering how much time I have left, how well I will live my remaining years, and whether this will be a state of joy, having meaningful relationships, good physical and mental health, sufficient funds to carry me through without facing financial difficulty, and continuing my contribution to the people and the world around me.

But what I am sharing in this book is more than my own experience—although without an intimate understanding of what it feels like, writing this book may never have been realized—but I also capture the essence of years of studying life, researching human behavior, and the secrets to living a fulfilling life.

What is that, you ask? It is a life characterized by lasting joy, health, wellness, and financial freedom. While you can incorporate many of the tips and tricks, the guiding steps to ensure continuous growth much earlier in life, midlife is an ideal time to make these changes to create a future you can look forward to with anticipation. Essentially, we define midlife as one characterized by creativity. This is when you may have much more freedom, financial stability, life experience, and stronger connections than when you first entered adulthood. Therefore, it is the ideal time to plan the rest of your life and change your course so that you can live longer and better. What I am going to give you are practical steps you can use to ensure that your life from here into your golden years is truly a time to celebrate, be at peace with, and, above all, enjoy.

Are You Ready to Have the Best Time of Your Life?

Are you ready to transform your outlook on your future? To learn about the Five Pillars of Longevity and how to strengthen them in your life? To be able to manage your stress far more effectively? Do you want to make the changes that lead to longevity and prosperity? To alter your perspective and allow inspiration, motivation, and creativity to shape your goals? Do you want to immerse yourself in daydreaming again, building castles in the sky as you feel everything is possible and within reach? Do you want to feel excited about the future again and look forward to the many tomorrows with anticipation?

Do I hear a resounding *yes*?

Then let's jump in right away.

1

LONGEVITY—IT'S PILLARS

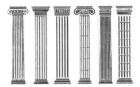

Life expectancy is a powerful and thought-provoking concept. Mostly because it carries a different emotional value for everyone. It is a term with deep personal meaning, leaving a different emotional response in us all. As this term contains the word *life*, it undeniably also refers to death, reminding us of our mortality.

For some, thinking about the term leaves them scared, concerned, anxious, or even stressed, while others are excited about the adventure lying ahead.

I've found that the most critical determining factor, whether you have a negative or positive perspective on your life expectancy, depends on how well you are prepared for life in its later stages. For many, the mere thought of life expectancy is enough to prompt them into action to ensure they enjoy life to its fullest. But unfortunately, others remain passive and almost locked in fear of not knowing what to expect.

Many factors influence life expectancy. Genetics, lifestyle choices, environmental influences, and medical advancements are most important. These are also the factors you need to address when you pursue longevity. However, before you do, it is best to gain a deeper understanding of the term longevity. You would also need to know what investments you would need to make to have a positive view on your life expectancy.

Longevity

The term longevity can be defined as enjoying a long life. A more scientific approach would define the term as the ability to survive life beyond average life expectancy (Longevity - an Overview | ScienceDirect Topics, n.d.). Understandably, many would consider longevity to be deeply desired. However, a longer life is only rewarding if it is also a good life. So, how do you define a good life?

Why Some People Live Longer Than Others

Soon, we'll take a comprehensive look at a wide range of factors that influence longevity. You'll have to address these factors in your search to live longer. Right now, my aim is to provide you with an outline of the top two reasons why certain individuals can anticipate a significantly longer lifespan compared to others. Many individuals have longer life spans without even making a conscious effort to do so.

Genetics

Do you come from a family where the average life expectancy is quite high or relatively low? Typically, those who come from a bloodline of people growing quite old have longevity genes that are quite effective in how they regulate oxidative stress. This is the stress of deterioration of your body on a cellular level linked to old age. So, if your family history reflects that many of your ancestors have lived long and healthy lives, you can already breathe a little easier. However, if the opposite is your reality, there is still a lot of hope for you, as genetics are only one major influencing factor.

Demographics

Living conditions are another major determining factor of longevity. For example, suppose you live in a pleasant, safe, and stress-free environment and have access to clean water, advanced medical care, and sufficient food resources. In that case, you are in a much better position than someone whose environment lacks all these amenities. But we can further break down the term demographics by looking at your culture, gender, and occupation.

For example, the average life expectancy for those living in Monaco is just under 90 years. The place has much sunshine, and they follow a largely Mediterranean diet, both serving as contributing factors to a long and healthy life. Other contributing factors are access to medical care, high food security, and a lack of adverse living conditions. (The 15 Places Where People Live the Longest, n.d.)

Then we can look at Lesotho. The African country has a life expectancy of only 56 for females and 50 for males and has the lowest life expectancy in the world (Countries with the Lowest Life Expectancy Worldwide 2022, n.d.). Contributing factors are adverse weather conditions, minimal access to health care, limited food availability, and lacking infrastructure. These are all contributing factors to a higher presence of disease.

The good news is that even if the odds are against you, you still have the freedom to make better choices for your future and to increase your longevity.

The Benefits of Longevity

The pursuit of longevity will demand transformation from you. Depending on the characteristics of your current state, these changes may vary between being merely challenging to downright hard. Unfortunately, change is often harder than expected, and you must be clear on your motivation for persevering with this transformation to maintain your rhythm along the way.

Therefore, before you even start making any changes, I would like you to determine why you want to increase your life expectancy. For some, this may be a desire born out of fear, but in the text that follows, I want to shift your focus to the many benefits you can enjoy from being successful in this quest.

More Achievements

How many goals do you still want to achieve in life? What experiences do you still want to enjoy? Where do you still want to travel? Do you feel that time is running out and you'll never be able to get to it all? Living longer and better gives you the time you need to accomplish your goals and increase your memorable life experiences.

More Skills

The more time you have, to learn and practice new skills to perfection, the more accomplished you become. It may be that you desperately wanted to learn a new skill during your younger years, but circumstances wouldn't allow it to happen as you had to obtain financial security, build your career, or raise a family. Now you can fit learning new skills into your schedule and have enough time to master them. For me, it was learning a new language, writing books, learning to play tennis, etc. What would you like to learn?

More Memories

The longer you have, the more things you can do or conversations you can have with the ones you love. Being at birthdays, weddings, or even attending graduations of younger family members can be a blessing many would love to have but simply don't get to enjoy.

More Opportunities

Do you still want to write a book, learn to paint, start a community garden, or expand on your legacy so that you can make a meaningful impact on the lives of those you leave behind? You may want to transform your neighborhood, and as you have the skills to do it, you would want to have enough time to be part of such an opportunity.

Better Medical Advancements

Today, healthcare advancements may be available that were still lacking a couple of years ago. Others may have passed away due to a disease that could've been cured with the medical care available now. Just imagine what medical solutions will be available 10 years from now or even 20. By making some changes, you can live longer and enjoy the benefits of better medical care.

More Enjoyment

Research indicates that happiness follows a U-curve. From about your early 20s, your happiness has been on a decline. However, this curve takes an upward turn at the age of 50, and you become happier as you age. Once you pass the age of 80, your average level of happiness exceeds that of those in their early 20s (Shrikant, 2022). So, the longer you live, the happier you become. Now, isn't that something to smile about?

What Determines Longevity?

The first step in the quest to live longer starts by identifying the factors that impact your life expectancy. You may find that you have little control over some of the factors determining your longevity. But there are many things you can still change to carve out a long and happy life. These things are enough to bring you the change you desire. We will explore techniques that will help you to enjoy longevity and the kind of life you may never have even thought you would be able to have. The changes you can make are so impactful that the factors you didn't have control over become almost irrelevant.

The Role of Gender

Just a few paragraphs earlier, I said that the life expectancy in Lesotho for women is 56 and for men is 50. This discrepancy isn't only exclusive to Lesotho. No, when we look at global statistics, there is a difference in life expectancy between the genders in every country. In Hong Kong, it is 88 years compared to 82, 86 against 82 for Switzerland, while Germany's numbers reflect 84 compared to 79. Men are always represented by the lower number. Globally, females have a longer life expectancy. There was a time when this difference was due to wars and men losing their lives on the battlefield. Today, the setting is somewhat different, and we can blame it on men predominantly filling positions holding greater risks while women are still underrepresented in many such workplaces. It can also be that men are fulfilling positions where they experience higher stress levels, are less equipped to manage stress effectively, or simply because men are more likely to exhibit risky behavior.

Hereditary Diseases

The top ten causes of death, according to the Centers for Disease Control (CDC), are heart disease, cancer, chronic lower respiratory disease, accidents, strokes, Alzheimer's disease, diabetes, pneumonia and flu, kidney disease, and suicide. Nine of these causes are linked to genetics, causing certain physical or mental concerns.

Prenatal or Childhood Care

Certain factors present during early childhood years or while still in the uterus can lead to lower life expectancy, even at advanced ages. Other similar factors can be caused by geographical factors impacting the quality of life during childhood. Both result in conditions and concerns later in life, causing a shorter life expectancy.

The Power of Education

Few students spending hours studying for exams or working on assignments would ever spare a moment to consider that what they are busy doing can positively impact their longevity (I am sure many of my former engineering students did not). However, research indicates that those who have completed a degree or any other form of higher education before they turn 25 increase their life expectancy. This is just less than two years for males, while females add almost three years to their lives. In comparison, the life expectancy of a man without a high school diploma is nearly 10 years less than his counterpart with a bachelor's degree (Beckman, 2016). These results are linked to the reduced likelihood of smoking and obesity in individuals with higher qualifications.

Getting Married

Weddings are a celebration of love and the moment you declare eternal love to your spouse in front of family and friends. This can also be a major step to increasing your longevity. Data shows us that married people outlive those who remained single or divorced. This phenomenon results from the fact that, generally, those in a committed relationship experience far less isolation and enjoy better heart health and longer-lasting mental health. In addition, being in a committed relationship motivates you to take better care of your health by letting go of unhealthy habits and going for regular health checks. Also, caring for other people around you and the responsibility involved may increase your desire for life and extend your life.

Ethnicity Plays a Role

There is nothing you can change about what ethnic group you belong to. Still, it is always good to be knowledgeable about typical health issues facing your ethnic group. This way, you can take steps to improve your longevity chances. CDC records indicate Hispanics have a longer life expectancy than non-Hispanic blacks

(Beckman, 2016). However, this is also linked to migrant work impacting the socioeconomic status of individuals.

The Socioeconomic Factor

Socioeconomic status is directly impacting life expectancy. This outcome is mainly due to the lack of access to proper health care, living in less-desired circumstances like high-crime neighborhoods, following an unhealthy diet, and in more severe cases, lacking access to clean water, to name only a couple of the factors impacting life expectancy linked to socioeconomic decline.

The Lifestyle You Follow

Your lifestyle either enhances or shortens your chances to live long and well. For example, suppose your lifestyle is characterized by unhealthy eating habits, eating lots of processed foods, a high alcohol intake, smoking, drug abuse, lack of exercise, or risky behavior. In that case, you will likely have a shorter life. The same is true if you are an adrenaline junky or have chosen a dangerous career path.

Access to Medical Care

Advancements in medical care have taken major strides over recent years. However, there are still many communities across the globe that can't afford proper medical care or, even worse, don't have access to such services. In these areas, the lack of medical care due to a shortage of medical staff, equipment, or prescription medication, reduces life expectancy tremendously.

Considering all the above factors, where do you place yourself when it comes to longevity? By determining your position, you'll have a much better idea of the effort and time you would need to invest in making positive change. However, even if several of these factors decrease your odds of living a long and happy life, it is not too late to change and turn around your situation.

The Five Pillars of *Living Longer, Living Younger*

A table standing on only one leg can be flimsy and topple over quickly. The more legs you add, the sturdier the table becomes. So, knowing that there are five pillars on which the pursuit of extended longevity rest is excellent news. But what are these five pillars on which your future rests, supporting overall health and wellness on a physical, mental, and emotional level?

Pillar # 1 - Eating Well

Food can fulfill many roles in your life, and there are different times when eating would resemble different things. Sometimes it is a way to pass the time. At other times food would be at the center of a celebration or a social event. Then there is eating to deal with emotional distress, and finally when you are hungry. While food can be important during all these events, it is vital to remember that the primary purpose of food is to provide your body with the nutrition it needs.

Any persistent shortages in your diet will lead to deficiency. This puts you at risk of medical concerns and diseases. In addition, overconsumption will cause weight gain or obesity, which is also at the root of many health concerns.

Balanced eating is founded on using your food as medicine and on supplying nourishment to your body. We'll cover nutrition in much greater depth later as a tool to care for your physical well-being.

Pillar # 2 - Remaining Fit

Far too often, we consider fitness and being active merely as ways to support physical health, and we underestimate its benefits to emotional and mental health. When it comes to exercise, it is important to note that you don't have to exert yourself with high-impact training. Instead, opt for moderate training that is sustainable, as consistency is the key when it comes to physical fitness regimes.

Pillar # 3 - Proper Rest

There is a myth that you would need less sleep as you age. This is a false belief, as the optimal number of hours of sleep you need remains seven to eight hours regardless of how old you are. Sure, some factors will impact your sleep quality as you grow older, but there are ways to address these concerns successfully to ensure that you still give your body the time it needs to recover and renew its cells.

Pillar # 4 - Stress Management

When you are experiencing high levels of stress, the body is persistently in a fight-or-flight state caused by an increased secretion of the stress hormone cortisol. There was a time when cortisol was considered a lifesaver. For example, in ancient times, our ancestors had to be on high alert whenever they left their caves. But now we know that unless you are experiencing a moment of imminent threat, cortisol is bad for your body.

Times have changed, and so has the environment we live in today, but the human body has yet to adapt to all of these changes. So, today we sit in a situation where our bodies experience the same response as if a saber-toothed tiger is hunting you down in a jungle, but unlike that scenario, the stress is not short-lived. When you experience a persistently high cortisol level, its impact on your health can be devastating. Therefore, effective stress management remains a vital pillar in supporting longevity.

Pillar # 5 - Social Connections

People are social beings, and having access to networks with strong bonds offers us the emotional support we need. Social interaction and connection become even more valuable to sustained health as we age. The confidence, joy, satisfaction, and sense of community we gain from social connections help prevent chronic disease.

These are the five pillars of longevity. Each point of discussion in this book links into these pillars in one way or another.

Lifestyle Changes

Living longer and better is not an impossible quest. However, achieving this goal does require that you make certain lifestyle changes. Depending on your current situation, these changes may be severe or minimal. Either way, it is important that you are consistent in the changes you make; therefore, it's better to opt for small but sustainable changes.

I'll cover these habits in much greater depth later in this book. But, for now, I want to give you a peek to spark anticipation by sharing how you'll have to invest yourself and the returns you can expect from making this kind of investment.

Establish a Healthy Diet and Rest Habits

I like to believe that nothing is impossible. It just depends on how much you want it. Being physically fit will go a long way toward ensuring that you live a long and happy life.

Coupled with that, getting enough sleep means seven to eight hours of shuteye every night. As you'll see later, the health benefits of sufficient rest far exceed what you can gain from that extra hour or two you choose to be awake. So, plan your schedule such that you have plenty of time to get the sleep your mind and body need.

It is also important to give your body the nutrition it requires, such as eating whole foods, plant-based options, reduced fat products (as long as it doesn't contain added sugars or artificial sweeteners), using less salt, and opting for fresh foods. It is best to avoid processed, calorie-dense foods containing minimal nutrients.

Avoid Things You Know Are Bad

If you know that something is bad for you, avoid it. Overeating, drug abuse, smoking, and drinking are all on the list of the most preventable causes of death worldwide. Every smoker I've ever met is perfectly aware of the dangers of the smoke they inhale every time they light up. Yet, they consider quitting to be a nearly impossible venture. That said, many people who have been smokers all their lives and then quit smoking confirm that, in hindsight, they can't believe it took them so long to quit.

Drug abuse and alcoholism may be much harder to give up as the withdrawal symptoms for both addictions can be quite severe. You'll find many resources, places, and professionals who can help you to beat your addiction.

Lastly, food and overeating. Often severe obesity is linked to emotional eating. If you are eating to soothe your emotions, I beg you to address these concerns. Then healing can start from within, and you no longer need food as a band-aid for your emotional wounds. As long as you allow old wounds to hurt you, you continue to empower the person who caused you injury. Choose life. Choose yourself and your happiness. Do what is necessary to quit the habits that can kill you.

Shed Unnecessary Stress

Stress is as much of a silent killer as the nasty and life-threatening addictions I've mentioned above. Stress is linked to some of the globe's most potent deadly diseases like diabetes and heart disease. It is undeniably linked to chronic inflammation in the body that can develop into auto-immune diseases and some forms of cancer. If you can't change your situation or move into a position where you'll be exposed to less stress, then increase your efforts to counter the impact of stress on your life. We will go into much greater detail about this too.

Seek Positivity

Studies indicate that a positive mindset can extend your life by almost eight years (Selig, 2022). That is a finding that is worthy of deeper exploration. After all, how hard can it be to focus more on the positive and less on all the negative in your life? The health benefits linked to being positive include lower odds of developing dementia. You'll also gain better hearing, balance, memory, and even the ability to walk faster.

Lack of awareness is the main contributing factor to a negative mindset. We are conditioned to focus on our worries about the future while our worst fears never materialize. If this is not the case, then we become mentally entangled in the regrets of the past, things we can do nothing about. How often do you find yourself just enjoying the present moment? The present moment doesn't have stress and contains no regrets. Be more mindful and cultivate a greater awareness of your surroundings, your sensations, and what is good about the moment right now. It is how you improve your general mindset from negative to more positive.

Once you become comfortable with being more aware, you'll take note of your thoughts and sooner notice when your mind is taking you down a dark alley of despair. You can then change your thoughts and try to sustain a positive mindset.

Define Your Purpose

What is your purpose today? Do you have a purpose that you've set for your future? A goal-driven life is a meaningful life and one with direction and intention. Unfortunately, many people merely float through life without having a set direction, like a rudderless boat on an ocean. Day and night, they are pulled around by the currents.

In comparison, someone with a purpose can travel a direct path despite the winds and currents. They can cover more distances in a shorter amount of time. What is your reason for getting up in the morning? What purpose would you like to fulfill in the next five years or more?

Ensure Financial Stability and Independence

Financial hardship has a way of pulling the carpet right from underneath your feet. The older you are when this happens, the harder the fall is and the more challenging it can be to get back onto your feet. Depending on your age, you might have been saving sufficiently over the past couple of decades and can continue the way you are, or you may have to be more money-conscious to be sure that today's expensive spoils don't spoil every day of your future.

Money is a major cause of concern and a valid cause of increased stress levels, especially if you are aging in a world that is experiencing an unfavorable economic climate. Explore your savings options and start investing more into building a financial cushion to secure your future dreams.

Love More, Be Kind and Compassionate

If you don't have a strong social network, start working on one now. If you don't have many friends you can rely on, start making more by joining groups that share similar interests. When expanding your social circle, aim to include greater diversity. Knowing people from different age groups, cultures, or social standing enriches your life and expands your mind. These friends will leave you feeling connected and positive. They help you overcome challenges with a fresh perspective and feel more secure.

These social connections also open an opportunity for you to contribute to the lives of others, leaving you feeling useful and like you made a difference.

Kindness should also spill over in the manner you treat yourself. There is no need to put the unnecessary strain of unrealistic expectations on yourself and accept that you will make mistakes. You are human too so learn to show yourself some kindness. The best way to start doing this is to note the things you say to yourself. Then determine whether you'll ever be as harsh to anyone else. If not, why are you so mean to yourself?

So, while there are many more steps to discuss, these seven steps or habit changes surely give you a lot to think about and incorporate into your life.

Let's Recap

The advances that took place over recent years made it possible to expect a much longer life span than only a couple of decades ago. Yet, while this is the case, there is still plenty you can do to help you become part of the population expected to live longer and better lives. So, are you ready to be a part of this favorable statistical cluster? In the next chapter, we discuss physical health and how you can ensure optimal longevity from the inside out.

2

IT STARTS WITH YOUR MINDSET

"Whatever distance you believe you can run is the exact distance you will end up running," (Crider, 2021). These are the words of seasoned ultramarathon runner, Michael D'Aulerio.

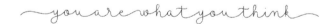

L ife is often compared to running a marathon, as it has many similarities with a long-distance race. Hence, we can borrow several life hacks from athletes participating in these long-distance races.

Athletes need to mentally prepare for such a race to have the mental endurance to continue even when every fiber in their bodies is screaming at them to stop. Likewise, you also need to invest time in mental preparation to increase your life expectancy.

What is your current prevalent mental state? Would you

describe yourself as a positive person who considers life wonderful even while facing challenges? Or are you more of a *glass-half-empty* kind of person? If you fall into the latter category, it is okay. It is never too late to learn to flip the switch from being negative to having a positive outlook on life.

What you focus on, you attract. What you attract becomes your reality. If you are fixated on your poor health, financial struggles, or deteriorating relationships, you will have more of this in your life. You are creating your own reality every day. However, most of us don't see it that way.

Coupled with this understanding is the following golden nugget—it is not the nature of your circumstances that determine your happiness but how you perceive it. If you are going to think that your life is terrible and you are always the one who suffers the most, then this is likely how your circumstances will remain. The same is true for thinking that your life is great and that you are extremely lucky to live the life you have. Then, you are likely going to enjoy increasing happiness and gratitude. The first time I realized this, it came to me like a life-changing revelation. In many ways, this truly is a life-changing revelation. It ultimately means that you are in control and can change your level of happiness in life.

If you are going to dread growing older and fear the day you become sick or so old that you lose your independence, you are already mentally preparing for unpleasant senior years. But you can also choose to look forward to this time of your life and focus on how great it will be, and you'll be far more likely to enjoy your golden years. The greatest obstacle to overcome remains uncertainty on how to make a mental switch from being predominantly negative to seeing life in all the hues of positivity and possibility.

Confronting Your Limiting Beliefs

It might appear that holding onto limiting beliefs is a way to protect yourself from rejection, failure, disappointment, or any other emotional consequence of your actions. I like to think of limiting beliefs as wolves in sheep's clothes. They come across as harmless ways to keep you safe. But in reality, these beliefs keep you hostage and prevent you from living to your full potential.

The Most Common Limiting Beliefs Linked to Aging

The following five limiting beliefs linked to growing older are quite common and are concerns that may be pressing on your mind too.

1. People will forget all about me when I grow old.
2. I will be less attractive when I grow old.
3. My time is running out.
4. Retirement is a time of extreme financial difficulty.
5. Gradually, aging will break my body down.

Can you list your beliefs regarding aging that may be holding you back?

Identifying Your Limiting Beliefs

Before effectively addressing your negative beliefs, you must determine what they are. Only then can you start to address them, setting yourself free from the power they have over you.

Are you ready to put your intentions into the effort and take the first step to live better and longer?

Grab a pen and notebook and list the limiting beliefs you have.

The following cues can serve as inspiration to get your mind going.

- I can't...
- I am too old...
- When I am old, I will...
- When I am old, I won't be able to...

You can fill in the blanks. For example, I can't just trust that the future will be great. I am too old to fall in love. When I am old, I will struggle to walk. When I am old, I won't be able to have fun.

Give your mind the freedom to identify all the beliefs holding you back from living your desired life.

The next step is to determine which beliefs have some truth hidden in them or are factual and which are mere figments of your imagination or false beliefs.

Putting Your Beliefs Through the Grinder

The best way to determine whether a belief is a fact is to question it as much as possible to see if it will continue to stand firm.

Take every belief you've listed and start asking questions about its validity. Of course, you need to be honest in your answers to enjoy this exercise's value. For example, if you want to question a belief stating that you will be forgotten when you are older, you have to ask questions like:

- Do I forget people just because they get old?
- Who are the older people I know who are still very relevant?
- What causes people to forget you? Is it really due to age?

- What can I do to prevent this from happening to me?
- Why do I think older people are forgotten?
- Are there other reasons, except age, that caused these people to be forgotten?

Once you've worked through all your beliefs, you'll notice many aren't real. So let go of those that proved to be merely present in your mind.

Replacing Your Beliefs

The best way to get rid of a negative or limiting belief is to replace it with something positive. You can find inspiration for your new, positive beliefs by looking at those you admire. If we continue with the previous example, you may look at people like Jane Fonda, Diane Keaton, or Jane Goodall. These women are all aging queens who remained relevant into their 80s. Remaining valid even at a mature age is relevant to both genders. I am referring to actors like Clint Eastwood, Sean Connery, and George Clooney, who all remained relevant at a mature age. Then we should also not forget most of our political leaders. Many of these people, whose choices often impact ours, are somewhat older (many are in their 70s and 80s).

Yes, their lives may differ vastly from ours, but we have one thing in common, we are all human. Are you convinced you can replace your negative belief with one that is more positive? For this example, I suggest a belief stating that the older you become, the more valuable your experience becomes to the next generation. Now, that sounds much kinder, doesn't it?

Change Your Course

Up until this moment, your limiting beliefs determined your actions. They served as the guiding light taking you through life. Now you've questioned your beliefs and could dismiss the false ones. You replaced them with positive beliefs, and your guiding lights have changed, and so will your actions. So, determine what steps you need to take to establish the influence of positive beliefs in your life. While you are at it, why not have a bit of fun while doing so? Just by being a little more daring in your actions, you will already enjoy escaping from the grip of negativity.

Change Your Crowd

We tend to surround ourselves with people who share our mindsets and beliefs. If you are primarily pessimistic, you've likely surrounded yourself with people who perceive life the same way as you do. If you are trying to change your mindset to be more optimistic, it is essential to put the people in your crowd under a microscope to determine who will weigh you down and prevent you from making the desired progress. It is very hard to stick to your plans if nobody in your circle shares your ideals, and it will be beneficial to befriend people who share the same positive approach toward life as what you are cultivating now. An inspiring way to do this is to pursue your hobbies and meet people who are excited about things that excite you.

The Power of Mindset

Changing your beliefs demands that you employ the power your mindset holds. But what does that even mean?

Defining Mindset

The word mindset is one of those words we use rather loosely in conversation without clarity on what it means. In its simplest form, the word mindset refers to the collection of all your beliefs about who you are and what you are capable of, but it also goes beyond that. Your mindset also consists of your beliefs regarding the world, other people, and their behavior. Therefore, it greatly influences how you experience life and perceive your future. In addition, your mindset determines your general attitude, reactions, responses, and interpretations of events and what others say to you. Can you see that if you want to change the quality of your life, you need to change your mindset, for it is what determines the quality of your life?

Two Types of Mindsets

We can divide mindset into two types: a fixed mindset and a growth mindset.

When you have a fixed mindset, you would typically believe that your talents, skills, characteristics, and level of intelligence are stagnant. But unfortunately, you don't realize the power you have to change these aspects of your being. Typically, people with a fixed mindset accept the hand they were dealt in life, and while they may not be content with their situation, they consider themselves incapable of changing it.

A growth mindset is far more powerful, and people who flaunt such a mindset are eager to improve. They know their abilities can be bettered through hard work and persistent efforts to establish change.

The simplest way to determine which category you fall in is to consider the typical behavior of people in each group.

Those with a fixed mindset would typically give up quickly. They don't see that their efforts bring about any results and therefore choose not to exert themselves. They are also the ones who would avoid challenges and risks. Feelings of failure often cloud their minds while they fear rejection or criticism. They don't like to celebrate the success of others as it leaves them feeling threatened. It is common for people in this group to have a scarcity mindset and to hold on to all they have, as the world has limited resources. As a result, they'll easily go through life without ever reaching their full potential.

This is not a favorable position to be in, and life as part of the other group is vastly more exciting, successful, and rewarding. In this group, you'll find people who love challenges, perceiving them as opportunities to grow and better themselves. It doesn't matter to them how often they fail. They continue to get up and persevere in working toward achieving their goals. They love to celebrate the success of others as they gain inspiration and motivation from those who succeed. Criticism doesn't hurt them as they consider it an opportunity to improve themselves. Therefore, they often live lives showcasing potential and achievement.

Can you see how influential your mindset is? It is one of the most significant factors determining your level of joy and satisfaction in life. Your mindset is a potent force to use to your benefit, and you have control over it to determine how you will apply it to your future.

. . .

Gaining Control Over Your Mindset Through Awareness

By becoming more aware of your mindset and its role in your life, you'll gradually gain greater control over your future, success, and finances and even gain more confidence.

Why do I say you have to gain greater awareness of your mindset?

Every single day of your life, your actions are determined by the thoughts in your conscious mind, but even more so by what is taking place in your subconscious mind. The significance of your subconscious mind is vast, and it controls roughly 95% of all your thoughts (Best, 2020).

Your beliefs and habitual way of thinking determine the decisions your subconscious mind makes.

Let me share an example of how the subconscious mind affects your quality of life. Denise and Jerry have been married for 25 years. They both recently turned 48. Denise is a teacher at a local school, and Jerry is an attorney at a small practice in the town where they live. Unlike their best friends who just got divorced, they are happily married. Until that one afternoon, Denise stopped at the mall to collect dry-cleaning and saw Jerry and his much younger secretary, Cindy, grabbing a coffee at the local Starbucks. First, she didn't know what to make of it, but she decided not to ask Jerry about it, as men always lie about their infidelity. Then her mind started to wander, and she remembered how their best friend's marriage fell apart when they turned 48 and how her friend, Sarah, blamed her husband's midlife crisis for all their problems. As time went by, Denise's focus shifted to seeking more proof that Jerry was cheating on her. Due to this increased stress level in their marriage, they suddenly started to argue over insignificant matters. The situation worsened until she told Jerry she knew he was cheating on her with Cindy. Jerry was blown away by his wife's accusation.

When Denise told Jerry what she saw, he immediately realized what was happening and asked her to wait. He went to his nightstand and came back with a little box. It contained a silver bracelet he got her for their anniversary coming up in two weeks. He explained that Cindy's fiancé owns the jewelry shop, and she went along to help him get a better price for the gift he bought Denise to celebrate their love.

Denise, who is usually someone who portrays clear thinking, was stunned by how her mind ran wild until she realized that her subconscious mind had taken control. It operated from her belief that couples are more prone to infidelity during their midlife. This is, of course, a belief ingrained in her mind during the many conversations she had with her friend, trying to support her during her divorce.

When you are unaware of what is happening in your subconscious mind, your mindset can take your entire life in a downward spiral and leave you feeling out of control. Through greater awareness, you can start to note what is happening in your mind and how it impacts your emotional state. It is when you can use your conscious mind to reprogram this negative way of thinking.

Using exercises like identifying your beliefs and questioning their validity, you can rely on conscious thinking to change your mindset and your subconscious mind's impact on your life.

Then you can start to change your mindset to work in your favor so that you can enjoy a positive outlook on life.

Mindset and Longevity

Let's cut to the chase. How long do you think you'll live? Don't get bogged down by thinking of all the factors you don't have control over. Instead, assume that these factors don't matter. Now, give the number of times you think you'll celebrate your birthday.

Yes, I agree that nobody knows when their last day will be. However, not knowing this date is a blessing in disguise. Can you imagine the severe widespread anxiety caused by every passing day, bringing you closer to *that* day? The unknown of your death date is also a way to encourage you to make the most of every day, as you never know whether it is your last day.

Nonetheless, research indicates that there is indeed a link between your mindset and how soon your days will run out. For example, a study published in 2017 determined a correlation between life expectancy and what is known as the failure mindset. When we look at the failure mindset in the context of aging, it refers to a frame of mind crippled by the fear of the consequences of growing old. Typically, those who suffer from this mindset have an overwhelming concern regarding losing control over their health, mental capabilities, and life in general. The researchers relied on the written works of several authors. They determined that those whose language has a negative tone—meaning they would often use words like helpless, fail, or any other term linked to failure—had a substantially shorter lifespan than those who don't use similar language. To ensure the accuracy of their findings, these experts continued to test the outcome against various factors impacting longevity, like demographics and the same birth year, and every time they came to the same conclusions (Zhavoronkov, n.d.).

What we can take from their study is that a negative approach toward life impacts your longevity.

While this is probably enough reason to transform your thinking from predominantly negative to more positive, I want to share another study with you.

In 1979, Dr. Ellen Langer took several men between the ages of 70 and 80 to a retreat for a week. The instructions were to enjoy life as if you were 20 years younger and to behave similarly. To make the experience even more real, she even used props to transform their environment to look like they were in the year 1959. She found that merely pretending like they were 20 years younger did these men so much good. They all appeared younger and enjoyed an improvement in their cognitive abilities, vision, and hearing. Needless to say, they were happier and looked and felt younger than when they entered the program merely one week prior (Barron, 2020). This demonstrates the extent of the impact of your mindset on the state of your life now and in the future.

Fostering the Right Longevity Mindset

You are most likely aware that your physical state starts to deteriorate when your mindset turns overtly negative. However, you also know that you feel much better after experiencing moments of joy. The studies mentioned above are an eye-opener to the importance of your mindset in determining your life expectancy.

Therefore, in our quest to identify the steps you need to take to live longer and better, we have to address the changes you need and can make to change your failure mindset into a longevity mindset.

A longevity mindset refers to the belief that you will likely enjoy a happy and healthy life and is linked to having a growth mindset rather than being stuck in a fixed mindset.

Avoid Blame

It can be easy to fall into a pattern of looking for someone or something to blame for everything wrong in your life. Avoid blame as much as possible, for nothing good ever comes from such an approach toward life. Rather than becoming fixated on all that is wrong or where you've experienced failure, focus on the positives in your life.

Avoid Comparison

Contrary to what those guilty of comparison believe, analyzing the similarities and differences is not a tool to improve yourself but rather a self-destructive way of thinking. You never have an accurate picture of what is going on in the lives of anyone else when you compare your likeness and the outcomes you enjoy with those of others. Yes, your neighbors may look like they have an amazing relationship with their adult children, but in reality, they are a family with many toxic secrets. Or how often have you felt inferior when you compare the car, home, or even clothes you can afford with that of someone else, unaware of the immense debt they have accumulated to have those riches while you don't owe anyone?

Unless you compare the version of yourself that you are today with the person you were yesterday, nothing good will ever come from equating your life with someone else. It is a sure way to spoil your mood and get you trapped in a loop of negativity.

Become More Mindful

As I've explained earlier, much of your thinking occurs in your subconscious mind. It means that negative thoughts can consume your thinking while you are allowing these thoughts to control your emotions, reactions, and behavior. Most likely, you aren't even aware of what is going on internally. This happens much quicker than you may think, as life can be so busy while your mind is consumed with meeting all your responsibilities that you are unaware of your internal state. Unfortunately, this state turns into the norm as time passes.

Therefore, you must become more mindful of your thoughts. Do so by regularly checking in to see what thoughts occupy your mind. Then, when these thoughts are negative and unfounded, gently nudge them away from you and think happy thoughts.

Increased mindfulness or awareness is the foundation of your efforts to improve your mindset.

Expect Failures

Life is the journey we take from our date of birth to the date of death. On a tombstone, life is represented by the dash between these two dates, a symbol that vastly belies its meaning. Nevertheless, this is all we have. During this time, you'll be making many mistakes and have many failures. However, you'll also enjoy vast successes and have many accomplishments to celebrate and be proud of. You choose which of the two you'll focus on, but when you make this choice, choose wisely. Ultimately, your choice will influence how far these dates are apart from each other.

Reflect Often with Kindness

Allowing time for reflection in your life gives you a chance to look back on past behavior and choices and how they impacted your life. Even more important is the opportunity to remind yourself of the lessons you've learned from your failures and how to improve them. But, of course, the same is true for your success.

Refrain From Attaching Too Much Value to Failure

Do you generally tend to obsess about your failures? People

portraying behavior linked to a negative fixed mindset tend to overreact to any insignificant failure. You are doing yourself an immense favor by accepting that failure happens to all of us as it is part of life but that it doesn't mean anything more than the value you attach to it. So, when you fail, consider it within the context of a much larger life, a life reflecting a lot of success too.

Celebrate Your Success

No achievement is ever too small to celebrate. Have you recently started art classes, and for the first time, you drew an apple that doesn't look like an orange? Celebrate the progress you've been making. Regardless of whether it is cutting 10 seconds off the time of your morning walk or finding what you're looking for online without any assistance, celebrate it. How you celebrate these accomplishments is up to you, as when it comes to celebrations, it is not how that is important but what it does for your emotional state and the sense of accomplishment it instills.

Let's Recap

Yes, your physical health, wellness, and fitness level immensely impact your life expectancy. However, even if you enjoy the most outstanding bill of health, it will all mean nothing if you don't have a positive outlook on your life expectancy. How you perceive aging remains the most influential factor determining whether you'll enjoy your golden years or be miserably trapped in old age.

3

THE SECRET TO HEALTH

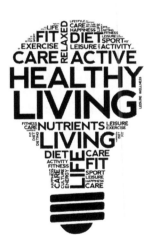

From the previous chapter, we can gather that much of the anxiety linked to growing older is caused by concerns linked to deteriorating physical and mental health. This is, of course, a valid assumption to make. However, from this stems the urgency to make the necessary changes to ensure a healthy lifestyle supporting your pursuit of a long and fulfilling life. In this chapter, we explore three of the most influential factors impacting your overall health and wellness: exercise, healthy eating, and getting enough sleep.

Move Your Body and Enjoy Longevity

Maintaining a healthy fitness level is beneficial throughout life, but increasingly more so when you grow older. With aging come several changes you don't have much control over. I am referring to your body's slowed production of various hormones, causing muscle mass loss and bone density. It is also a stage linked to a slowing metabolism causing increased weight gain, which can cause several serious health concerns.

While you may not stop this from happening to your body as you grow older, you can slow down the process, and getting enough exercise is one of the most effective ways to do that.

But how much exercise is enough?

Any effort to increase your activity level is better than doing nothing. So, if you are leaning toward being more of a couch potato, even taking a stroll in your neighborhood or getting into gardening is already progress. However, the ideal activity level for those 65 years and older is a minimum of 150 minutes of activity per week. You can break this into 30 minutes per day for five days of the week or two sessions of 75 minutes each. It depends entirely on what works best with your lifestyle and schedule. Keep in mind that this should be at least moderate exercise. The term moderate indicates that you'll still be able to hold a conversation, but there should at least be some sweating. Examples of moderate exercise are hiking, running, jogging, or even brisk walking.

That is not all, however. To fight off the loss of muscle mass, you should also include strength training two days a week. Building your core muscles is a necessity as we age. Another concern older people have is the loss of balance. Simply standing on one foot and holding your balance for a couple of minutes about three times per week will help you do that. Make sure you lightly support yourself against a wall or use a chair to start. Yoga and tai chi are also helpful ways to improve your balance and reduce the risk of having a nasty fall.

While exercise improves your balance, protects your muscle mass, and supports bone density, it also supports your cognitive functioning. As you switch between tasks while exercising, you are not only giving your muscles a workout but also protecting your brain cells from decline-causing concerns like dementia and Alzheimer's disease and other similar concerns.

The last benefit I want to share is more complex and is linked to telomere health. Telomeres are the caps located at the end of your DNA strings. Throughout your life, they gradually grow longer, but when they grow too long, they keep your cells from dividing, a process necessary for cell regeneration. When this happens, the odds of high blood pressure, heart disease, and strokes increase substantially. Studies indicate that the telomeres in older people who have been predominantly inactive are much longer than in the ones who are pretty active. While there is still uncertainty about how it happens, the mere fact that exercise is confirmed as an influencing factor is already enough reason to get active (Seegert, 2021).

I want to take these benefits one step further so you can see how enjoying the health benefits I've shared practically impacts your life.

Improving your balance prevents falls that often lead to severe injury and a painful recovery. This is a topic I expand on in much greater detail in my book *Never Fear Falling Again*. If you suffer a fall, the likelihood of getting a fracture decreases, and the speed at which a fracture will heal increases if you have better bone density. Exercise improves your flexibility and strength, making it easier to move around. Through mobility, you'll enjoy greater independence. Once older people become entirely dependent on others, they often feel isolated, leading to depression. So, while taking a brisk walk in the park may appear insignificant and a waste of time, it can be the determining factor in ensuring your independence and longer life expectancy.

What Type of Exercise Should You Do?

Many different types of exercise will ensure a range of health benefits. For example, aerobic exercises like running, walking, and swimming increase your fitness level and improve your heart health. These activities also improve lung health, forcing your chest cavity to expand. Another tip is to choose scheduled activities with a group or team commitment. This will add to your motivation to participate regularly.

For strength training, safe and trusted options are squats and bicep curls. If you are doing these exercises for the first time, it is best to start slow. Initially, you may not need weights to get a great workout in, but as you become more fit, you may want to start using weights gradually when you are training. Always take care not to overdo it, for you may take a bit longer now to recover from any form of injury than 10 or 20 years ago.

For improved balance, standing on one leg and tai chi will suffice, but you can always explore more options as your fitness level increases. In *Never Fear Falling Again*, I cover several helpful steps and tips to improve balance. Improving your balance might appear to be an insignificant goal, but preventing this fear from taking over your life is an effective solution. It is a way to keep your independence and remain socially active.

Exercising Safely

Exercising safely should always be your primary concern. Therefore, please don't start with any exercise regime if you haven't checked in with your doctor first. This is especially important if you 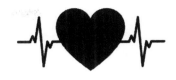 have any underlying health concerns or are on chronic medication.

Take it slow at the start. If you overdo it in the beginning, you are exposing yourself to injury. Even when your fitness level has already improved significantly, it is still crucial that you always listen to your body to prevent injury. Be sure to follow the directions for the exercises and increase repetitions gradually.

I completely support the idea that sometimes you must push through even though you don't feel like it, but there is no need to injure yourself and end up stuck with pain or discomfort. If your body needs a break, take that break, but do return to your regime when you recover.

Except for taking it slow when necessary, you can also prevent injury by wearing the right clothes. For example, wearing the wrong shoes when walking or running can cause muscle spasms and other injuries.

Always warm up your muscles before starting, and remember to take it easy toward the end. Stretching your muscles when done will also reduce stiffness and pain.

Make sure that you have enough water to keep your body hydrated throughout.

Don't Have Time to Exercise?

Do you struggle to see where you'll fit daily exercises into your already overburdened routine? Don't fret, as you are not alone. It can sometimes be hard to know how you'll work in a new activity, especially if you are not keen on doing so. The good news is that the fitter you get, the more your body will crave this activity, and the more you'll enjoy it. Until you get to this point, increase your activity by making a few minor changes during your day. For example, take the stairs rather than getting into an elevator or take a walk rather than your car. You can also use these moments to multitask. For example, a brisk walk with your friend can turn into a quick chat and catching up on what is happening in each other's lives, or a short jog with your dog means it has been for a walk too.

Keeping Going When the Going Gets Tough

Often, when you start something new, like taking up an exercise regime, the first couple of times are easy to partake in as you are still highly motivated and inspired. But what happens when the motivation and inspiration fizzle out? Then you need to have specific fail-safe steps in place to ensure you keep up your fitness regime.

The following tips can be beneficial here:

- Pick an activity you like and that excites you (have you tried pickleball? :))
- Choose something that fits into your routine.
- See if you can make this a fun activity too, like dance classes with a friend.
- Choose something that doesn't require a huge capital investment before you start.

In short, when you increase your level of activity by choosing a fun activity that interests you, maybe something that is close by and doesn't require you to travel far to partake, or something that is socially enjoyable and doesn't require much of you to start, it is a much more sustainable option for you.

Healthy Eating

Increased activity will vastly improve your life expectancy, but it will be even more effective if you couple it with healthy eating.

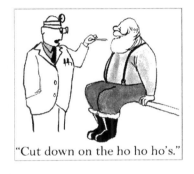

"Cut down on the ho ho ho's."

Essentially, you become what you eat, and if you are hooked on unhealthy, overly processed foods, it will eventually show. Food may play one of many roles in your life. Sometimes it is at the center of social events and friendly gatherings. At times you may eat out of boredom or to seek emotional comfort. Yet, the primary purpose of food is to provide your body with the nutrition it needs to sustain itself. With this approach toward food, food becomes your medicine, and your need for prescription drugs will decrease.

A diet that supports longevity contains a lot of food in its most natural form, lots of raw fruits and vegetables, and whole foods like legumes, whole wheat products, lean meats, and healthy fats and oils. These options are nutrient-dense and low in calories and salt content.

Some excellent options to include in your diet are:

- **Cruciferous vegetables.** Have some brussels sprouts, broccoli, cabbage, or kale to help your body detox itself. These vegetables are high in fiber and extremely nutrient-dense.

- **Berries.** Berries are high in antioxidants. Including berries in your diet will also help to improve your brain health as it reduces the impact of aging on your cognitive functions. There is also a link between eating berries and reduced blood pressure and cholesterol levels.
- **Pomegranate.** This is a one-of-a-kind fruit with a sweet-but-tart flavor. Some health benefits linked to this fruit are cancer prevention, heart health, and improved brain health.
- **Legumes.** Beans, peas, lentils, and chickpeas are all high in fiber and therefore prevent constipation, improve blood sugar levels, and are even linked to preventing colon cancer.
- **Turmeric.** The golden spice often found in curries is loaded with antioxidants and plays an important role in cell renewal, delaying aging.
- **Chia seeds.** Chia seeds are nutritious and are another source high in antioxidants. They are linked to lowering the risk of heart disease and improving blood sugar levels.
- **Green tea.** Green tea improves brain health, and can prevent type 2 diabetes. It also plays a role in preventing several cancers.
- **Walnuts.** These nuts contain a variety of minerals that contribute to brain health. They are high in antioxidants and help to prevent heart disease.

These foods are some of the healthiest options you can choose from to help you fight off health concerns linked to aging.

However, while some foods are great to include in your diet, several food types are best to restrict to the minimum or, even better, avoid altogether.

- **Sugar.** You don't need to include any additional sugar to your diet as your body gets enough energy from the sugar in fruits and vegetables, as well as the carbohydrates found in whole grains.
- **Red and processed meat.** Animal protein can be hard to digest and does place an unnecessary burden on your digestive system. However, red meat is also high in fat content, contributing to excess weight and increased cholesterol levels. Processed meat is also high in fat, but also contains high levels of preservatives that turn into toxins as well as salt.
- **Alcohol.** In small quantities, some types of alcohol can be beneficial. For example, red wine can contribute to your health. That said, it is important to limit your intake as most types of alcohol are high in empty calories. Then you also need to consider the strain you place on your body, contributing to faster aging when it has to process and clear itself from alcohol.

Food to Fight Inflammation

As mentioned earlier, food has healing power, and by including certain foods in your regular diet, you can combat a range of health concerns linked to growing older. In addition, by doing so, you are supporting your goal of longevity. For example, when your body is exposed to chronic inflammation, you are more prone to developing autoimmune diseases such as celiac disease, multiple sclerosis, and Addison's disease. However, inflammation also causes a greater vulnerability to develop certain cancers. Adding the following foods to your diet gives your body the nutrition it needs to clear up and prevent inflammation.

- sweet potatoes
- ginger
- turmeric
- olive oil
- fatty fish like tuna, salmon, and mackerel
- fresh fruit
- squash
- anti-inflammatory herbal teas

Food Supporting Brain Health

Do you fear the day when you walk into a room and can't remember why you went there in the first place? Or looking for your car keys and not knowing where you put them down last? Maybe it is forgetting names that scare you the most and the fear of having to introduce someone and not being able to remember their name.

These are all quite normal signs of aging that most people experience. Losing your memory is not the same as dementia or Alzheimer's disease, but it can be frustrating and affect your confidence. As you grow older, certain parts of the brain—the areas where learning and more complex mental activities take place—gradually shrink.

Blood flow toward the brain also slows down, keeping it from getting the nutrients and oxygen it depends on. Added to that, aging also affects the communication between nerve cells.

Do understand that these are all normal changes to expect as you grow older. But you can still take action to slow down the effect of aging on your brain health. The simplest way to take control of this situation is by including foods that support brain health in your regular diet. For years, many people have enjoyed lasting memories simply through effective diet management.

The following foods support brain health:

- broccoli
- blueberries
- avocado
- fatty fish
- whole grains
- sunflower seeds
- dark chocolate

I understand that knowing what food you need to eat and what you should avoid can be confusing. However, constantly thinking about what you must have and what can harm you can become such a daunting venture that you may want to throw in the towel. Therefore, instead of working on portion sizes or the nutritional value of every food type you eat, opt for a healthy way of eating, like the Mediterranean diet.

The Mediterranean Diet

This specific diet is the common way of eating around the Mediterranean Sea. As residents enjoyed lasting health and wellness, their way of eating became a point of interest across the globe. Lately, this way of eating has turned into a highly recommended diet supporting longevity.

Researchers have found that a specific way of eating reduces heart disease and the chances of having a stroke. It also contributes to lowering the risk of cancer and stress's effect on the body and improves the odds of not getting type 2 diabetes. Other benefits are that it supports bone density and brain health. The latter results from several recommended foods that contain high levels of omega-3 fatty acids (Williams, 2022).

The Mediterranean diet includes most of the foods already mentioned and typically consists of more legumes as they are high in B vitamins, iron, and antioxidants. You can have meat, but in small quantities and not every day. It also restricts your alcohol intake and limits sweets and sugary products. Make sure you consume these foods in raw form, but when you use oil for cooking, it should be higher-grade olive oil. You can also drizzle olive oil over your vegetables or on salads.

Intermittent Fasting

Fasting is an ancient practice often linked to religious observance. However, fasting allows for specific times during the day when your body doesn't have to digest food and can take care of cell renewal and generation, combating aging.

You can follow several intermittent fasting (IF) methods. The most popular choice, as it is easy to sustain and convenient to fit into your busy schedule, is the 16:8 fasting method. It entails that you'll fast for 16 hours and have an eating window of 8 hours. A rough guideline is that after 10 hours of fasting, the glucose level in your blood drops to such a low level that your body must turn to alternative energy resources. This is when it starts to burn fat, which is a more stable and cleaner energy source. When this happens, your body enters a state of ketosis, meaning it now relies on fat for energy, contributing to weight loss. Still, you also enjoy several other health benefits.

While intermittent fasting is an easy way to ensure optimal calorie management, there are also several other benefits you can enjoy.

- It allows your insulin levels to drop, preventing insulin resistance which is the cause of type 2 diabetes.
- IF helps to increase the levels of the human growth hormone (HGH). HGH plays a vital role in preventing the loss of muscle mass.
- Cellular repair takes place much faster, meaning shorter recovery from injury or disease. Through this process, your body also clears itself from toxins much faster.
- Even certain genes experience changes leading to greater longevity (Gunnars, 2021).

The topic of IF is quite vast, and I expand on it in much greater detail in my book *Intermittent fasting: Beginner's Guide To Weight Loss For Men And Women Over 50.* I urge you to read up more on the topic as it is single-handedly one of the best choices you can make to improve your quality of life, even at an older age.

By combining the Mediterranean diet with IF, you place your-self in an optimal position to enjoy all the benefits both diets offer. In addition, this is an easy way to ensure accurate calorie manage-ment while having complete guidance on what food to include and what to abstain from.

When it comes to eating, it is essential to remember that every-thing you eat does impact your health in one way or another. The older you get, the greater this impact is. Yet, there is always time to make the necessary dietary changes to reverse the aging effect of years of unhealthy eating. It is also important to remember to eat *slowly* and cherish every bite. Many experts tout the benefits of mindful eating.

The Power of Sleep

How we underestimate the power of sleep is a matter of wide concern. We are a society that often spends minimal time sleeping as we are hooked to screens until late at night. Whether you are binge-watching your favorite series or reading a book on an electronic device doesn't matter. The blue light you are exposed to keeps your brain from shutting down and preparing for restful sleep. But what benefits do you miss out on every time you get out of bed after insufficient sleep?

While you may be sleeping, your body is hard at work. This is typically when it diverts all its resources to care for cell renewal and repair. It is when your body goes through a complete restoration of all cells that were damaged in your body, including skin cells. Do you have bags underneath your eyes when waking up tired? Or do wrinkles seem to increase drastically after having several days of insufficient sleep? These symptoms indicate that your body doesn't have enough time to take care of cell renewal. Did you consider the term beauty sleep to be merely a myth? It is indeed while sleeping that your youthful appearance is restored.

The influence of sleep goes much deeper than the surface, however. While you are sleeping, your brain is also busy storing memories. During this time, it processes all the information gathered during the day. Therefore, a lack of sleep causes a lack of focus and impaired cognitive abilities. It will also increase toxin levels as there is not enough time for the brain to clear itself from the toxins accumulated during your waking hours. These toxins are harmful to your brain. Therefore, it is no surprise that a persistent lack of sleep is linked to Alzheimer's disease (Tennessee, n.d.).

Then there is also heart health to consider. A lack of sleep is directly related to increased blood pressure impacting your heart health. If you are persistently missing out on vital sleeping hours, you are increasing the risk of type 2 diabetes, as this will affect your insulin functioning, causing high blood sugar levels. Disrupted sleep also impacts your immune system and makes you more vulnerable to disease.

Can you see how a lack of sleep contributes to many health concerns linked to old age, making it a significant concern for longevity?

As you grow older, several factors influence your quality of sleep. The number of times you may have to go to the bathroom at night will likely increase. Frequent urination is one of the most prominent disruptions of quality sleep.

Other factors include changes in your circadian rhythm, experiencing pain and discomfort, and changes to your sleep patterns —such as becoming a much lighter sleeper causing you to wake up often, and then having trouble falling asleep again (Tennessee, n.d.).

Tips to Enjoy Better Quality Sleep

For the longest time, bedrooms had only two purposes. It was a place for making love and sleeping. As computers turned into laptops and mobile devices found a place on our nightstands, bedrooms became a place where you could also catch up on work. This notion may be convenient, but it is destroying your mental connection with your bedroom, which is a place of rest. Is this the case in your home? You will benefit from putting an end to this habit. Instead, consider your bedroom as a place to relax, where you sleep.

It will also help to set a sleep routine in place. It can take some time for your brain to wind down and be ready to fall asleep, and you can speed up this process by following the same routine every night before going to bed. Once you start this routine, you are already sending signals to your brain that it is time to sleep.

Going to bed at the same time every night is another way to establish this routine.

Limit the number of times you need to go to the bathroom by cutting down on your fluid intake an hour or two before going to bed. As you age, your body may also become more sensitive to substances like caffeine. If coffee keeps you awake at night, limit your caffeine intake to mornings only. Having a heavy meal late at night, or at least close to bedtime, can also negatively impact the quality of sleep you enjoy.

Are you napping during the day? Having a nap can be a real treat, but it can also be why you struggle to fall asleep at night. Limit these naps and see if you experience an improvement.

How active are you during the day? Most jobs require employees to sit at a desk for hours with little activity. If you are in one of these jobs, you need to find other ways to increase your activity (take the stairs, park at the parking spot far away from the building, etc.). By increasing your activity level, you will also improve your sleep quality.

Stress and anxiety caused by excessive worrying are other factors that can interfere with your sleep. While it can be hard to let go of your worries, it will help transform your bedroom into a peaceful environment. Soft lighting and soothing music can be helpful aids. In addition, many apps today will provide background sounds, naturally reducing your anxiety levels to help you fall asleep.

I mentioned your circadian rhythm earlier on. This is your body's natural rhythm, going from active and alert during the daytime to being at peace and ready to rest at night. This rhythm is primarily impacted by your exposure to sunlight. Older people often don't spend as much time outside and get exposed to daylight as they used to when they were younger. This can also affect your sleep quality. Make a point to spend some time outside or take a melatonin supplement to get the relief you seek.

Lastly, read a book. The emphasis here is on a book in paper form (a print book) and not an electronic version illuminated by light which will keep your brain waves active. Transporting yourself to another time and place through a good story can provide comfort and replace day-to-day worries.

Let's Recap

How you perceive aging greatly impacts your life expectancy, but your physical state is even more influential. Most of your fears about growing old are linked to your health. In this chapter, I explored that by being more active, committing to healthy eating, and getting enough sleep, you can drastically reduce the odds of getting any of the much-dreaded health concerns linked to aging. These steps may appear insignificant, but as you've just learned, poor management of either can ripple out and put you at risk of developing several health concerns threatening your longevity. While these concerns can all impact physical and mental health, stress is the biggest threat to lasting mental wellness. In the next chapter, we will explore the impact of stress and how you can reduce its impact on your life to lengthen your life expectancy.

4

MONITOR YOUR MENTAL HEALTH

Let's talk about Mental Health

F ar too often, the topic of mental health is considered taboo, as if we are not allowed to discuss our mental health in the open. Added to that is the understanding that mental health only refers to severe concerns like being bipolar or even schizophrenic. In this chapter, I am stepping away from this perspective as mental health also refers to the state you wake up in every morning. Or what your mood is like during the day, your overall enjoyment and contentment with life, and just how happy you are. I am sharing tips on how to effectively live a life that still includes stressors, as these tips will help you manage stress better.

Life can be complicated at times. The nature of life and the obstacles it throws in our way is just one of those things we have to overcome. So is stress. We live in a modern society structured in a manner that makes it nearly impossible for ordinary men or women to escape this stress. Yet, here too, you are not merely a hopeless victim who needs to play the cards you were dealt. You can learn new skills or master your existing techniques to manage stress effectively. Excessive stress over a long period can affect your mental health, impacting your quality of life.

Mental Health and Aging

The biggest concern regarding mental health is that most people still do not prioritize health and wellness. Yes, we are taking significant strides to improve this situation globally, but is it enough? When was the last time you thought about your mental health or whether you are taking care of yourself in this regard?

The statistics paint a gloomy picture as the World Health Organization informs us that those suffering from severe mental health concerns can expect a life expectancy shortened by 10-25 years (Hull, 2022). That is an intensely concerning number. The impact of such a concern divests in many ways and eventually leads to a higher likelihood of chronic and infectious diseases. It increases poverty, causes poor self-care, and in extreme cases, can lead to homelessness and even suicide.

Destress!

It doesn't matter how we look at it—there is only one effective way to overcome the impact of stress on our lives—we need to destress. You are probably already painfully aware of your need to destress, especially during the hours when you should be asleep but are staring at the bedroom ceiling with only your thoughts to keep you company. Yet, that is not all there is to it. A Yale research study concluded that while stress is a known factor leading to strokes, heart attacks, and even diabetes, it also makes you grow older faster (Perkins, 2022). Furthermore, compared to the study participants who failed to manage their stress levels, those who did manage stress effectively remained mentally and biologically younger. In short, it means that the effects of aging were more severe in those who were unable to manage their stress.

If you are unfamiliar with the signs of stress, it can be easy to oversee how badly it is already impacting your life. Typically, you'll become irritable, anxious, or nervous when stress shows up in your life. As a result, you may struggle to find any joy in life, even when doing things that would typically make you happy. Nothing seems funny anymore, and you are shaded by a constant cloud of dread. These symptoms eventually cause you to lose interest in life and dread every day. You may even feel lonely or neglected, not to mention that you, too, will start to ignore those things that used to matter to you.

As your mind and body are so interconnected, stress impacts you on a physical level too. Excessive sweating, trouble sleeping, constant fatigue, itchy skin or rash, digestive problems, and even muscle pains are all linked to stress. Then, of course, the worst experience is suffering a panic attack. Even if you still manage to have a long life, is this the kind of life you would want to live, feeling this way all the time?

The Causes

What causes you to feel this way? Many reasons can cause or contribute to stress. These causes vary from bills that are heaping up to health scares and broken relationships and can truly be unique and stressful for everyone.

When we consider stress, we must recognize that there are two types of stress. Eustress can be used to obtain a positive outcome. Have you ever met anyone who believes the stress they experience is what propels them toward their success? They are the ones who would wait until just before a deadline hits them to start working. Eustress is a manageable form of stress. You'll find it in all kinds of scenarios at work, at home, and in your relationships. It is the kind of stress that pulls you right out of the complacency in your comfort zone to grow and better yourself.

Then there is also distress. This is the type of stress leaving you feeling disempowered, overwhelmed, and, quite frankly, often sick to the stomach. It doesn't contribute to your life in any positive way and is extremely harmful to your mental and emotional health.

The way to tackle distress effectively is to destress.

Introducing Guided Imagery

Guided imagery is an easy technique that doesn't require much time and will leave you feeling less stressed and much more relaxed, and as a result, you will notice how all the other stress-related symptoms in your life also start to disappear. Technology makes it so easy for us to enjoy the benefits of such techniques, as there are many apps that are often completely free, offering you the guidance needed without even having to step out of your home. Some of the most used examples of these apps are *Headspace, Calm,* and *Breethe.*

Some may consider guided imagery as a form of meditation, but it can also be described as a deep form of relaxation. You can choose how much time you have to spare for a guided imagery session and turn to this solution as often as needed. It merely requires you to find a peaceful spot to lie down or sit relaxed and undisturbed.

It will be helpful to get an app on your smartphone that you can listen to as it will guide your mind, or you can also decide to zoom your focus and thoughts onto one pleasant place or scenario.

While your mind is consumed with negativity and stress-provoking thoughts, it continues to release stress hormones into your circulation. The primary purpose of these hormones is to put you into the fight or flight mode and protect you by making you more capable of defending yourself. However, the cause of your stress is only present in your mind and isn't real. As a result, you'll continue to feel stressed as the situation you are physically prepared for is not real and, therefore, can't be resolved. The result is that as the human body is perfectly developed to benefit from short bursts of the stress hormone, the effect of persistently high levels of these hormones in your blood can be detrimental. It is when you can feel your body tense up and all the other symptoms of stress present themselves.

Through guided meditation, you recreate a similar effect, but this time around, you focus on positive, feel-good things, allowing your body to relax as the level of cortisol and other stress hormones decline. As a result, you'll gradually become more relaxed and revitalized and feel positive and energetic.

Guided meditation is one way to approach stress and better manage it. Another is progressive muscle relaxation.

Progressive Muscle Relaxation

Let's get practical. I'll share the steps, and you can try progressive muscle relaxation before we continue. This exercise could take anywhere from 3 to 10 minutes, depending on how quickly you proceed.

Again, you'll have to find a place to sit or lie down without being disturbed. I recommend lying on your back as this will make the exercise really easy. Close your eyes and breathe deeply. Then, start at your toes and lift your toes (without moving your feet) toward the ceiling before stretching them forward. Repeat this a couple of times. Then move onto your feet and ankles and tighten your muscles before gently letting them relax. Continue the same process for your calf muscles and knees, then move to your hands. Squeeze and release your fingers, arm muscles, and, eventually, your shoulders. Continue squeezing your buttocks, lower back, upper back, and abdominal muscles. Always squeeze, pause, and relax. When you reach your head, purse your lips, wiggle your nose, open your mouth wide, and relax again. Even your eyebrows can do with a lift and then letting go. When you've worked every muscle from the tips of your toes to your crown, you can end the session with a couple of deep breaths before getting up.

This was a session of progressive muscle relaxation, a technique promoted by an American physician, Edmund Jacobson, to improve your mental health through an approach to relax your muscles. It is a widely applauded method to relieve muscle pain and anxiety and to improve sleep. If you struggle to fall asleep at night, try this in bed and see how your sleeping habits improve.

Here too, you can rely on technology for assistance. Again, great apps to download on your smartphone are *Calm* and *Headspace*, but you can also try *Happify* and *Breathe2Relax*. Another excellent resource in this regard is *Spotify*, where you'll find many options to choose from.

More Options to Destress

These shared methods are great ways to manage stress effectively, but there are many other forms of destressing to consider. You can even rely on a combination of techniques to achieve the desired results, an outcome that will support your quest for longevity.

Acknowledge Your Stress

You can only start working on improving any challenge or concern once you've admitted it exists. The longer you deny that you are stressed, the longer it will take you to take the necessary steps to manage it better. So, stop suppressing your stress and accept that you are overly stressed and not managing it, and then take action.

Change Your Approach Toward Stressful Situations

I've said it before and am doing so again. Any situation is exactly how you perceive it to be. The same truth is valid when it comes to stressful situations. If you are going to dread these situations and fear their existence in your life, you will likely perceive the situation in a much more stressful manner than if you accepted it as part of life. You always have the choice to see things in a different light. Just think about a situation that is a major concern for you. How can you change your perception of this situation to remove the fear and anxiety it provokes in you? For me, the best approach is to ask what is the worst that can happen. Then, if I am prepared for the worst, the situation somehow seems less daunting, and usually, my worst fears never come true.

· · ·

Accept—Choose—Act

If there is one technique that highlights how much power you have to manage your stress instead of allowing it to manage you, then it is this technique. Accept—Choose—Act (ACT) is a trusted method where you can accept your stress factors. You can choose how you want to manage them and then also how you will act to overcome them. So, you can accept what you are dealing with, and the fact that stress is part of life. You then choose in which direction you want to proceed and how you see your life progress beyond this obstacle. Lastly, you take action to bring about the change you desire and to continue realizing your goals, in this case, pursuing a long and happy life.

Aromatherapy

The scents and aromas at the center of this kind of therapy have proven effects on the brain and brainwave activity. It is amazing to know that simply by surrounding yourself with the right scents, you can reduce the level of stress hormones in your body, slow down your brain's activity and feel how your body and mind slowly relax. Burning candles or scented oils, bathing with essential oils, and using diffusers are all ways to destress yourself passively.

Hug Someone

Regardless of our differences, there is one thing that connects us all. Our human nature includes the need for physical touch. While a comforting touch during a moment of distress does wonders to calm you down, there is also proof that when you get hugged by a loved one, your brain increases the secretion of oxytocin. This hormone lowers blood pressure and stress hormone levels, creating instant relaxation (Scott, 2022). So, if you need a hug, ask for it. It is a caring act that results in mutual health benefits.

Take Time Out

You need a break from time to time. We all do. Being constantly busy increases your sense of being overwhelmed. It will also lead to exhaustion, and even the most superficial concern can come across as overwhelming when you are tired. This is why it is so important to schedule time for leisure activities. These activities —such as reading, sports, and socializing—help you refocus and rejuvenate. As you derive so much pleasure from these activities, they lower your stress levels and make you more resilient to handle stressful moments. Whether you immerse yourself in arts and crafts, gardening, or baking doesn't matter. It should only be something you enjoy doing.

Yoga

Yoga is an ancient form of relaxation but also much more. Yoga consists of a light exercise to stretch your muscles, but it is also a form of meditation, helping you relax and become better at managing your stress. There are several forms of yoga you can explore to find the type that best suits your lifestyle and personality and relieve your stress.

Be Grateful

Expressing gratitude is one of the easiest and most effective ways to overcome the impact of stress. It is a process that demands you shift your focus away from all your problems and concerns to all that is good in your life. It is also a way to remind yourself how many resources you can access to overcome obstacles, making success more achievable. You can set time apart to think about all you are grateful for or even start a gratitude journal where you can keep a record of all you are thankful for.

Stress Journals

Another form of journaling you can choose to include in your life is keeping a stress journal. Journals remain safe places to vent and get rid of negative emotions and energy without offending anyone. You'll also find that simply putting your stressors into words will already bring about a great sense of relief, and you'll be able to find the solutions you seek.

Take a Walk

Sometimes the best way to get the distance between yourself and a stressful situation is to walk it off. Take a quick walk to get fresh air. The activity will increase your feel-good hormones. Putting distance between yourself and the situation will also help to gain a different perspective on the matter. So, rather than staying in a place that increases your stress, take 10 or 15 minutes and walk around the block. If you can take this walk in nature, it is even better as nature enhances the calming effect.

Take Care of Your Relationships

Many of the concerns and fears linked to growing older are linked to isolation and loneliness. A lot is written about the importance of a strong network of relationships, especially during your older years, as these relationships provide you with comfort and are your support structures. They also create opportunities to be socially active, contributing to lower stress levels.

Eat Well

You might be familiar with how your food impacts your physical health. However, it does influence your mental health too. So always take care to include food that will provide you with sufficient levels of B vitamins and omega oils, as these are all hugely beneficial in your goal to improve your ability to manage your stress well.

While each of the tips I've shared will improve your overall ability to manage your stress, combining these steps in some fashion will prove to be an even more effective approach to stress management. However, there is something else you can also do to take care of your mental health. I am referring to preserving your cognitive functioning.

Preserve Cognitive Functioning

The term cognitive functioning refers to a range of mental abilities like learning, memorizing, understanding, reasoning, and intuition, to name only some of these vital functions impacting your overall 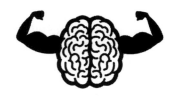 ability to remain independent and content in life. There are several reasons why these abilities decline over time as you age.

Typically, this kind of decline shows itself as being more forgetful, losing your train of thought midway through a conversation, or struggling to find your way in an environment you are familiar with. It can also cause judgment errors or feeling over-whelmed more often.

There are several factors contributing to cognitive decline as you age. It may be due to chronic medication you need to take to manage another health symptom or due to hormonal changes. Vitamin deficiency is also a concern linked to this kind of mental deterioration. When your blood chemistry experiences change in sodium, calcium, or even glucose levels, it can have a similar effect on your cognitive health.

These are all causes that can occur gradually. However, more abrupt changes in your cognitive ability may result from injury, substance abuse, or exposure to toxins.

As your ability to remain highly functioning is crucial to enjoying a longer and happier life, I wanted to share some techniques and tips to help you preserve it for as long as possible.

Cognitive Stimulation Therapy

As retaining a high level of cognitive functioning is essential to growing old successfully, cognitive stimulation therapy might be the solution you seek. This kind of therapy will have greater relevance to you if your family history shows that your genetics may cause advanced cognitive decline.

Cognitive Stimulation Therapy (CST) is a short-term treatment option used to improve the symptoms of those experiencing the impact of dementia or Alzheimer's disease. This treatment has effectively slowed the process, especially in those experiencing mild or moderate symptoms. While CST is used as a therapy to treat those whose mental health is already declining, it is also a great way to preserve cognitive functioning in those who are merely growing older.

CST is presented by a qualified professional in either individual or group sessions. Often, it will require that participants focus on certain memories like childhood events, and from these memories, a deeper discussion will flow. Another approach would be to encourage conversation over more relevant current events. In many cases, these therapy sessions may even take on a more practical approach. For example, they can include activities like throwing a ball or completing a creative group project.

Reversing the Impact of Cognitive Decline

While CST has shown itself as a highly effective approach to remedy the impact of cognitive decline and slow down this decline process, there are alternative steps you can take to prevent or slow down the deterioration caused by aging before it becomes so severe that you need CST.

Most activities that require creative thinking, speaking, writing, or problem-solving will keep your brain active and serve your brain health, like exercising would help your body. There are several fun ways you can include this type of exercise in your day.

Puzzles

Spending time completing puzzles is one of those activities people can either take or leave. Some enjoy the relaxation they find in letting their minds focus on nothing but getting the correct pieces to fit together. Others would never consider puzzles worthwhile and have no interest in doing them.

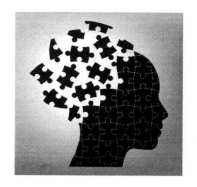

Regardless of which group you identify yourself with, your cognitive functioning will improve from this activity. Puzzles offer an effective exercise to improve brain function and mental capabilities.

It is also important to include crossword puzzles under this umbrella term, as these, too, are great for exercising the brain.

Sudoku

Sudoku is designed to improve problem-solving skills. It is an affordable way to exercise to improve your cognitive skills. However, don't underestimate the positive impact of accomplishment on your mental and emotional state when you finish one of these number puzzles.

Board Games

Later, I will explore the benefit of social interaction and how this serves as another way to preserve your mental health. Board games are fun and create an excellent opportunity for social interaction. It is a great way to make beautiful memories with your children or grandchildren and is the perfect excuse for spending time with friends.

Learn a New Language

When you stop exercising a muscle, it becomes weak. Initially, you'll experience a deterioration in the muscle's effectiveness, which continues to decline until it loses all or most of its abilities. The same is true for your brain. Your career might have changed, you may have retired, or you are no longer mentally challenged. These factors can cause you to no longer use certain parts of your brain, and this will cause them to decline. Learning a new skill, especially a new language, will give your brain the necessary workout. Learning a new language is highly challenging, but it will keep your mind sharp.

Reading

It is widely known that reading more often keeps your brain active and in great shape. It doesn't matter what genre of writing tickles your fancy. Just giving your brain exposure to new ideas, perspectives, or even a peek into the lives of others, is an effective way to improve your cognitive functioning. If you don't have the time to sit and read, then listen to an audiobook as you walk or go for a long drive.

Crafting

Have you always been a creative person? Maybe you have wanted to spend more time being creative but have yet to get around to it. Now is the time you can immerse yourself in such activities, give your creative energy an outlet, and push your brain beyond its comfort zones. Creative activity demands your brain to be resourceful as you create something out of nothing, but it is also a fantastic way to relax and eliminate any excessive stress.

Getting Active

Again, we've explored how your physical health can benefit from being more active, but this kind of activity will improve your mental health too. Activity that will speed up your heart rate will ensure that more oxygen and nutrients are carried to your brain, providing it all it needs to remain in optimal condition. As exercise requires moving around, it also exercises your alertness and combats mental fatigue. Finally, aerobic exercise will improve your circulation, and spending time in nature (while you exercise) is calming to the mind and the soul.

Improving Your Social Life

Regular social activity is another way you can improve cognitive functioning. The benefits of having an active social life will impact your mental health in even more areas. Numerous studies indicate that those who maintain strong social connections and meaningful bonds enjoy greater longevity (An Active Social Life May Help You Live Longer, 2019).

These benefits are rooted in the fact that by being socially active, you avoid facing the impact of isolation on your mental and physical health. Isolation is linked to a decline in immune function and increases the risk of premature death by as much as 50% (An Active Social Life May Help You Live Longer, 2019).

There is, of course, another way to look at socialization and how it contributes to longevity. At the beginning of this book, we touched on widespread fears related to aging and loneliness. Feeling isolated is one of the top threats to enjoying a long and happy life. Feeling lonely increases your stress levels, but the idea of being lonely has a similar effect. Therefore, you can dismiss this fear by ensuring you have strong social networks. These social networks will also provide emotional support when needed, and the deep bonds you will form with others in this network will add purpose to your life.

The Three Most Influential Social Connections

We can divide social connections into three categories. We all have these connections, but to determine the state of your social life, it will be helpful to consider each type of relationship individually.

First up are intimate connections, referring predominantly to those you love dearly. In this category, you'll usually find family and friends. You consider yourself to be very close to these people. Relationships with people of different generations can be normal in this group and may happen automatically. For example, if you live with your children and grandchildren or have regular contact with them, people from different age groups will be present here.

The second category is called relational connections and refers to people whom you regularly see, like work colleagues, fellow patrons at your church, or perhaps the parents of the friends your children made while at school. In this group, you'll also find people like the waiter who regularly serves you at your favorite restaurant, your pizza delivery guy, or even the cashier at the nearby convenience store.

We can refer to the last group as the group of collective connections. In this group, you'll find people you've met at the club where you are both members, volunteers committed to similar passions for helping out as you, or even the parents who serve on the school board with you.

Do you have strong bonds in all three categories? Can you identify what brought you together to form these bonds, and what sustains the health of these connections?

The Antidote to Loneliness—New Friends

When you were still a child, making friends might have been easy. However, this becomes harder as you age. I often hear people express uncertainty about where to find new friends. Even though you may not realize it, there are still several places where you can easily make new friends with people who will support you when you need it.

Join a Club

In my opinion, clubs are the easiest way to make new friends. There are so many choices to pick from. What are your interests? Maybe you are into dancing, reading, or even a specific sport. These clubs all offer you the chance to meet like-minded people who share your interests. Therefore, it is easy to make conversation, even if you are more introverted.

Friendship Apps

We live in an age of technological advancements, and there are apps to get almost anything you desire, from romantic partners to friends. Friendship apps enjoy growing interest as these platforms are great for making acquaintances that can become good friends. Another platform you can use is to join specific groups on social media platforms. These also offer you the chance to meet new people and get to know them to a certain degree before ever meeting them personally.

Explore Your Neighborhood

What is happening in your neighborhood? How involved are you in your community? Simply by venturing beyond the parameters of your property, you are likely to find many people who have at least one interest in common with you, your location, and maintaining the standard of living it has to offer. Many exciting projects are running in various communities where you can get involved and meet new people who can, over time, become your friends.

Get Out

There are many ways to make friends, but there is one sure way you will stay in isolation—simply by never venturing out of your comfort zone. The reality of life is that you have to go at least halfway to meet new people. So, step outside and visit your local park, museum, or even the beach or a nearby lake. You'll find plenty of people who will likely respond favorably if you start a conversation. Even if you are not making new friends in such an environment, spending time amongst people will surely leave you feeling less isolated and lift your spirits.

How to Deepen these Bonds

Now that you know all the possible ways to meet new people, you can progress to the next step, deepening these bonds. Making friends is a process. First, you need to meet new people and decide whether you want to pursue a deeper friendship with them. There are several tips for strengthening these bonds once you've determined that you like someone enough to pursue such a relationship. Eventually, the power of socialization to enhance mental health is not nestled in the number of people you know but in the quality of bonds you have with them.

The best bond-building tips are:

- **Ask good questions.** Most people like to talk about themselves and if you allow them to do this and you show genuine interest in what they have to say by listening actively, they are bound to feel connected to you too. Ask questions about their interests, their family, or even what they want to achieve. It is usually best to refrain from sensitive topics like religion or political viewpoints until your bond has become much stronger. It is also important to remain aware of the fine line between being interested in what they have to say and being intrusive with your questions. However, even while considering these two no-nos of initial social interaction, there is still a lot to talk about.

- **Look your best and be confident.** Before stepping out of your home, consider how much value you attach to the appearance of others. Now, look at yourself in the mirror and see if you look like someone you would want to meet. If not, it may be time for a wardrobe change, haircut, or investing in your appearance in whatever way necessary. By feeling good about how you look, you will radiate confidence. Confidence remains an attribute that attracts the interest of others.

- **Look for the good in others.** Yes, you need to look good, but you also need to look for the good in others. Rather than being fixated on the many ways you differ from those you meet, shift your attention to all you have in common and how much alike you are. Seek the good in others and it will become much easier to befriend people with whom you can form meaningful bonds.

- **Show that you care.** Helping someone is a great way to grow the bond you have with them. This is even more so if they didn't expect you to lend them a helping hand. If you listen carefully to what they say, people will share their concerns and challenges and if you can offer assistance, do so without expecting anything in return.

- **Maintain an open mind.** The world is much more diverse now than ever before. In your venture to expand your social connections, you are bound to meet people of different cultures and backgrounds. Keep an open mind and be ready to learn from them. This is the kind of contact that will enrich your life and make your life enjoyable, and of course, these are also the kind of connections that contribute to longevity.

Let's Recap

I think most of us have witnessed someone much older than ourselves who was perfectly capable of living a full life physically, but somewhere during the aging process, they got a mental health diagnosis that is robbing them from enjoying life. Witnessing such suffering can be fear-provoking. It is normal to worry about your mental health when you consider growing older.

Yet, there is always time to make a couple of changes to improve your odds of the same happening to you. First, reduce your stress, as stress is poison for your mind. Exercise your mental muscles with CST or any other fun activities I shared. Second, start forming strong and meaningful bonds with people you like, even if they differ vastly from you, and allow their presence to enrich your life and offer support when needed.

Next, we are addressing ways to overcome another huge threat to longevity and looking forward to this time in your life: financial health.

5

WANT TO LIVE TO A 100? YOUR FINANCES MATTER TOO!

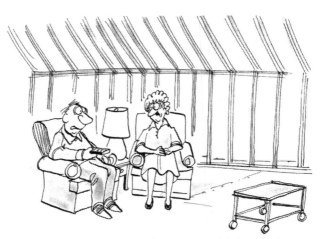

"Those were years of such ambitious plans
... before the money ran out."

I am sure you know that money can't buy you happiness, but it sure comes close to it, and the lack of sufficient funds can rob you of your joy and satisfaction. Unfortunately, this is a scenario that only worsens as you grow older. While you are still earning a salary, you at least have the comfort of knowing that there is still an inflow of funds into your account, even though it may be a slow trickle, barely enough to cover your expenses. But once you are retired, the situation can worsen if you didn't plan for the day you no longer have an income.

Then we also need to consider that the purpose of retirement has shifted quite a bit over the past decade or more. Retirement is no longer limited to only those who have reached a certain age. Instead, in our modern society, far more people choose to retire earlier in life as this gives them the time to pursue their passion and to do what they've always wanted to do, may this be to pursue a mere hobby or to turn this hobby into a new income stream.

Are you planning for your retirement? If so, are you ensuring you have access to sufficient funds? In 2022, the CDC stated that the current retirement age is around 62. The life expectancy for Americans is set around the age of 79, while you are likely to be part of the large group of people who get to have even more birthdays (Segal, 2023). Will your money last long enough to be financially secure for the rest of your life after retirement?

This is a question that keeps many people across the globe awake at night. While limited funds for old age can already paint quite a dire picture, even worse is when your situation takes a turn for the worst, and your health deteriorates, or any unforeseen matter sucks you dry long before the time you expected your funds to last.

Financial Planning for the Future

Sadly, the picture I had to sketch was not pretty. It is normal to feel your stress levels increase if you can identify with the situation. But let's take a step back and inhale deeply, for it is not too late to change your situation.

Saving Matters

The odds that you are still in your 20s are slim—I haven't had the pleasure yet to meet many 20-odd-year-olds concerned about longevity — but even if you are, I need to emphasize that it is never too early to start saving for your retirement. However, it is also never too late to jump into action if this part of your future planning is lacking behind.

In this chapter, we will cover several solutions on how you can make up for the possible deficit in your future finances.

Retirement planning is essential because:

You don't know what the future holds for you. Most people only consider their future living expenses according to what it is at the moment. However, life can become far more expensive if you include chronic medication or specialized treatment or care into your budget. It might also be that it is not your health that deteriorates but that of a loved one, and their medical care can be expensive. It is one of those cases where you would rather be over- than underprepared.

Simply knowing that you've made sufficient provision and are financially secure enough to remain comfortable even when challenges arise is an immense stress relief. The stress over financial concerns can be so severe that it puts your relationship or marriage under unnecessary strain.

In light of poor retirement planning, you may be making even more mistakes. By putting proper measures in place to save up for the future, you'll be able to cut down on the taxes you are paying. By getting adequate guidance from a trusted professional, you will be gathering sufficient funds to take care of the future and be able to pay Uncle Sam less.

Always remember that every choice you make today regarding your career and income will impact your future. So, always focus on where you are heading and the impact of your present decisions on your future financial security.

As someone who unexpectedly went into early retirement, I know how scary it can be. It is a turbulent time in anyone's life, but the sting of this happening becomes less painful if you know you are properly financially prepared for the future. In my case, I was offered a generous early retirement package that I could not refuse. The cash I received as a part of this package allowed me to spend the time to develop my other interests and engage in activities that brought me additional income.

Take These Eight Steps!

Let's assume you find yourself in the worst-case scenario and have no financial planning for your retirement. Simply following these eight steps will help you progress in the right direction. Even if you have some planning in place, these steps will still allow you to determine how well-prepared you are and if you are making sufficient financial provisions for your retirement.

Determine Your Current Financial Standing

What is your current net worth? Many people are so fixated on their monthly paychecks that they have no idea what their net worth is. Simply add up the value of all the assets you own. The list will include things like your car and house, any investments, and the money you have in the bank. Now, calculate all your debt. Here we are looking at loans, credit card debt, student loans, if any, your mortgage, and any other money you may owe. Subtract the sum of all you owe from the sum of your total assets, and the answer you get will be your net worth.

Increase Your Worth

To be more financially secure, you need to have a greater net worth. There are two ways to increase your net worth; increase the value of your assets or reduce the value of your debt. For now, let's focus on growing your net worth by increasing the value of your assets. Next, consider how you can increase your income. This may be through making a career shift to access a higher salary, investing your savings to earn interest, starting a side hustle, or getting a passive income.

Determine How Much You Would Need for Retirement

Many say that the most challenging part of financial planning for the future is the self-discipline needed to save. I beg to differ. The most challenging part is to prepare for an uncertain expense. There is no foolproof way to determine precisely how much money you'll need to enjoy a comfortable retirement. There are so many factors beyond your control that can impact your situation. We can look at concerns like unexpected changes to your health, disasters, and global finances plummeting again. The list is too long and anxiety provoking to include all here.

My advice is to talk to retirees. They are the people who have experience with the situation you are preparing for and will be able to give you much greater clarity on what to expect. From this information, you can determine what your net worth should be to enjoy a carefree retirement.

Find the Right Retirement Plan for You

Next, you need to do your homework to determine what retirement plan options are available and then weigh the pros and cons of each to see which will be best suited for your life now and in the future. I am no financial advisor and recommend that you seek the help and support of an expert in this regard, but soon I'll give you an overview of what options are available.

Educate Yourself on Money Matters

Studying finances may be something you have little interest in. Still, we have a responsibility toward ourselves and our loved ones to educate ourselves enough to understand what we are investing in and whom we trust with our money. After all, you've worked hard for all you have, and the person who'll take the best care of it is you. So, read up as much as possible about finances and current trends, and learn some commonly used terms. Simply put, become money smart.

File Your Will

Suffering the loss of a loved one is already extremely disturbing and disrupting life, but if your loved ones also have to deal with financial uncertainty, life can become truly hard for them. Drafting and filing your will is the responsible thing to do. When there is a will in place, settling your estate and ensuring your loved ones are still cared for is the responsible thing to do.

Identify a Retirement Side Hustle

Often large corporations have a set retirement age. When you reach that age, you need to let go of your monthly income. If you are sure your savings aren't enough, it will be beneficial to start working on your side hustle. This is a great way to increase your net worth, and I've even come across retirees who are now making more money from this than they did while working full-time. Getting the right side hustle can be a lucrative way to secure your financial position.

Revisit Your Plans Regularly

Times change, and so do circumstances. Therefore, revisit your plans regularly to determine any changes in your current net worth and future finances and see if you need to adjust your plans.

The Best Retirement Plans

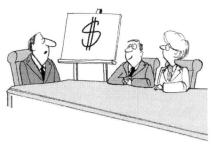

"Great plan. Could we get some more details?"

The good news is that you can choose from several retirement plans. Even though I am not a financial advisor, and you should discuss your choices with an expert in retirement planning, I want to give you an overview of each option.

When considering your options, remember your goals and risks and how much time you have left until retirement.

Defined Contribution Plans

Defined contribution (DC) plans are the best-known type of retirement financing option. They are so popular that until recently, up to as many as 86% of all Fortune 500 companies only offered these (Royal, 2023). This is also the larger group of financial plans in which 401(k) plans fall—more on these next.

What is important about DC plans is that they limit employee contributions to $22,500 per year. This number increases annually and is much higher for those above 50, where the limit increases to $30,000 annually. Getting a DC plan is a great start, and it is also good to know that you don't pay any taxes on this money until you start withdrawing from it.

401(k) Plans

The most significant advantage you'll enjoy from 401(k) plans is that the money you invest into retirement this way isn't considered part of your taxable income. Thus, you enjoy tax savings by adding funds to a 401(k). In addition, these plans make saving easy as you can schedule your deductions, and by the time you withdraw your funds, your withdrawals will be considered in the same light as any other form of income. However, while you may have these funds sitting there, you will most likely have to pay a penalty if you access them earlier for an emergency. You are also restricted to how much money you can put into a 401(k), so if you want to put more away for your retirement than stipulated, it is best to add another option portfolio.

· · ·

Individual Retirement Account

An individual retirement account (IRA) is the answer the US government had to help Americans save for retirement. The plans limit contributions to $6,000 for those younger than 50, while those above this age can contribute $7,000. These numbers are also adjusted over time. There are different types of IRA plans.

Traditional IRA plans offer brilliant tax benefits like not having to be taxed on these funds until you withdraw them. These investment vehicles can also allow you to invest in stocks, real estate, or bonds. But here, too, if you want to withdraw some of these funds in advance, you'll have to pay taxes and penalties. Other options in this category are Rollover IRAs, Spousal IRAs, Roth IRAs, and SIMPLE IRAs.

Traditional Pensions

If you are employed, this is a way to save for retirement that requires minimal effort. You would have a fixed monthly benefit, and therefore, you reduce the risk of your money running dry before you die. The con of this saving solution is that the size of your benefit is linked to the number of years of employment. So, if you started at a new firm not too long before retirement, the benefit amount can be very small. Furthermore, it is a savings option that is dying out as the number of companies offering this benefit is declining (Royal, 2023).

Guaranteed Income Annuities

A common way to increase your retirement savings would be through guaranteed income annuities (GIAs). Here you take complete responsibility for your savings investment. GIAs offer monthly payments and are considered an additional income stream. However, if you are still determining when you will retire or even planning on retiring, you may need to get greater clarity on your plans before investing in this option.

The Federal Thrift Savings Plan

This can be an option for you if you meet the requirements of being either a member of a uniformed service or of government. If you proceed with this option, you'll have a choice of five different investments, including an international stock fund, a bond fund, or an S&P 500 fund. The benefits are that you'll be viable for a 5% contribution from your employer, which is only one of a few more small contributions you can benefit from. The most significant risk of this savings option is that you have no guarantees regarding the size of your available balance when you retire.

Cash Balance Plans

This solution is similar to a pension plan, but where a pension plan pays out funds, these plans offer contribution and investment credits. The benefit is that you will have a relatively accurate idea of what you'll receive. Still, if your company makes any changes related to its pension solutions, you risk losing out. This is also a solution that will only be truly beneficial if you've been working for a substantial time for one employer.

Cash-Value Life Insurance Plans

This is a solution offered by several companies and is more than merely a retirement plan option. You can also gain death benefits from this solution and the cash benefit that can add to your retirement solutions. So, essentially, you'll be financially protected against several risks, but if you slip up on this and your policy lapses, you will have to pay quite a bit of taxes. Therefore, these plans are better suited for people who are already somewhat financially secure and only want to add to their retirement funds when all other options have run dry.

Nonqualified Deferred Compensation Plans

In short, NQDC plans are mostly limited to only a segment of the population already financially secure. The plans offer a way to reduce taxes, but they aren't great on promising security as if the company turns insolvent, your funds will be drained too.

Free Yourself From Debt

Ideally, you would want to settle all outstanding debt before you retire as this will leave you feeling more secure. However, we all know that sometimes life happens, and things don't pan out as planned. Then you may very well end up with debt that needs to be settled after retirement. While this is not a favorable position, it is also not a life sentence. The following tips will help you eliminate your debt and free yourself from its burden.

Stop Making More Debt

If you continue borrowing money, your efforts to become debt free will be futile. So, stop making any more debt. The most common—and easiest—way to make more debt is by swiping your credit card for all those unnecessary purchases. If you can't take control of your spending, cut up that card and protect your financial state.

. . .

Minimize Overall Spending

The reality is that your income may have reduced quite a bit after retirement. However, you aren't broke. But, if you don't align your expenses with the income you receive from your retirement options, you will most likely find yourself in an unfavorable financial position that may be very hard to recover from. Therefore, you must cut down on spending and live a simpler life.

Downsizing Is an Option

Do you still stay in your large family home even though the children moved out years ago already? Large properties generate higher monthly expenses, and essentially you are paying for things you no longer need. Sure, when you were raising your kids, you wanted to have a well-kept garden, and you had the income that made it easy to maintain your property, but now you don't need this space anymore, and you may benefit from downsizing.

Settle Only One Payment

When you have multiple sources of debt, it can be hard to keep up with all the payments you have to make. It may also be harder to settle your debt as there is the constant interest added to the outstanding amounts every month. So instead, consolidate all your debts and then make one payment. When you've chosen this option, you are also more likely to get a better interest rate, making it easier to settle the entire amount.

Consider Credit Counseling

When your outstanding debt is adding too much stress to your life, you will likely benefit from reaching out to a credit counselor.

These professionals have the experience to help you to get rid of your debt step-by-step. As this is a free service, you won't have to pay any funds to the company offering this assistance, and you will be able to enjoy the comfort of having a plan to get rid of your debt.

Applying for Bankruptcy

This may be the last option you want to choose, and nobody envisions their golden years having to undergo such a process. Yet, there are times when this may be the best option to get rid of your debt.

When you file for bankruptcy, your social security funds usually remain protected. If you aren't a property owner, this can be a much more attractive solution than what you may initially think. However, if you do file for this, it will reflect on your credit records for as long as 10 years, preventing you from borrowing money any time soon.

Consider an Investment Portfolio

Pension funds and retirement plans aren't the only ways to make provisions to have enough financial security to live long and happily. No, you can also start or expand on your investment portfolio. Typically, when you are older, the best options to settle for in this regard are investment options that offer minimal risks and higher returns. Unlike investors who started to build this portfolio in their 20s or 30s, you may have a much shorter timeframe to generate maximum returns from your investment. You also don't have time to risk losing any funds as there will not be enough time to recover from such a setback.

. . .

It would be best if you considered the following investment options.

Certificates of Deposits

This investment option secures your principal amount— which is a good thing as you will never be left with less money than what you've invested—and you'll get a fixed annual rate for as long as your money is invested. The rate may vary from time to time, but you can also choose to lock in your interest rate at a set amount. The benefit is that you can be sure of getting a specific amount of interest, but if the rates increase to above what you've locked yourself in, you will be making less than you could have.

Individual Stocks and Bonds

This type of investment may demand that you have at least a basic understanding of how stocks and bonds work to ensure that you make smart choices that will bring you the returns you need on your investment. Options you may want to consider are:

- **Bond ladders** as they improve the risks of investing in bonds. Bonds offer lower risks but also be aware that they are more susceptible to changes in interest rates. Bond laddering will entail that you invest in several bond options which will all mature at different times. Through this method, you'll be less likely to have to sell earlier and have a more accurate idea of what your cash flow will look like.
- **Preferred stocks** are considered to be a priority when a company becomes bankrupt, meaning this option is low-risk. This investment option will also not give you

any voting rights but you will see higher and even more consistent dividend payouts.

- **Low-volatility stocks** are the answer to getting more out while facing fewer risks. Traditionally when you consider investing in stocks it is the case of how higher the risks you are facing, the bigger the returns will be. When you choose to invest in low-volatility stocks, you will still enjoy relatively good returns without the risk. These stocks have also proven themselves in the market as a favorable investment option.
- **Dividend stocks** have fund managers taking care of your stocks on your behalf, making it an investment option that doesn't require as much work or a perfect understanding of the stock market. Dividend stocks pay out funds periodically and can be a great passive income stream.

60/40 Portfolio

Let me start by saying this is a wonderful option if you want to invest your money but not your time to learn the basics of trading and investing. It is an entirely hands-off investment approach, and your portfolio can include bonds and stocks. Once you've found a broker who understands your needs and concerns, you can trust the investment part into their capable hands.

This investment option offers a fair blend of risks and returns, making it profitable without losing sleep over the risks. It doesn't mean, though, that the option is entirely safe, as there is always the possibility of having a combination of increasing interest rates and inflation, causing the value of stocks and bonds to fall. However, the risk is still a worthwhile one to take.

. . .

Annuities

If your biggest fear is outliving your money, annuities might be your solution. You can expect a never-ending income stream from this kind of investment. The con to this solution is that buying annuities can be pricey. Therefore, when you do, be discerning and only choose options that will answer your needs.

Investing in Funds

There are several types of funds you can invest in, like index, mutual, and exchange-traded funds. The best approach would be not to put all your eggs in one basket, so diversify your portfolio to balance out the risks and rewards of each of these options.

Real Estate as an Investment

Real estate is a wonderful solution to generate a passive income. Once you've invested in a property that is not your primary home, you can rent it out and generate a rental income from it or opt for short-term leases. The latter is generally a more lucrative option if your property is in a prime location. Just be aware that short-term rentals can deliver a seasonal income. However, they are also usually more labor-intensive to take care of.

Budgeting for Retirement

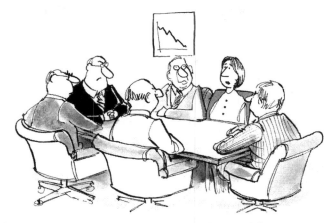

"So much for counting on a lottery ticket to capitalize the retirement fund."

One of the first steps to ensure that you are financially secure during retirement is to estimate how much money you would need to retire. Now, I want us to explore how you can budget your expenses during retirement to have complete certainty that you know where your money goes.

The following five steps will guide you as you prepare your plan:

1. Determine your income by adding up all income streams that provide you with a steady cash flow, as well as the total of all regular expenses and determine the total amount you are left.

2. If your expenses are too high, divide your expenses into three categories namely, essentials, nonessentials, and seasonal expenses. Under essentials, you'll list expenses like groceries, accommodation, clothes, and transport costs. Nonessential expenses usually include

travel expenses, gifts, and membership fees. Seasonal expenses can be rather large expenses, but they aren't due monthly. For example, your car's registration, taxes on your property, and even birthdays or Christmas can fall into this category. When you have clarity on where your money goes, it will be easier to cut down on these expenses.

3. Health care can become an unexpected and expensive expense, so always leave room in your budget to put additional money aside to carry you over during such a financial challenge.

4. A budget is only effective if you manage it properly. Therefore, you may have to push yourself to be more disciplined in your spending to ensure that your funds don't run out before the end of the month.

5. Test your budget to see if it is a practical solution. Before you reach retirement, it may give you greater peace of mind to live according to the budget you've drafted to see if you need to make any changes to your plans. The best time to do this is while you still have an income so that you can see how effective your plans are.

Remember that even if your budget is working well and you stick to it perfectly, you will have to regularly revisit this plan to see where you can improve or need to make changes.

Before we move on to the last chapter, I want to conclude all I have to say about financial planning by sharing a bit more about the 4% rule.

Exploring the 4% Rule

Are you familiar with this rule linked to retirement planning? The 4% rule states that, during the first year of retirement, you can withdraw as much as 4% of the value of your retirement portfolio. While having $100,000 set aside may seem unrealistic, it will provide us with a simple example of how this rule works. So, during the first year of your retirement, you can withdraw 4% of this money, meaning you can withdraw $4,000.

During the second year of retirement, you may have to consider inflation. If inflation is set at 3%, you can withdraw the amount allowed during the first year plus inflation. So, you can withdraw $4,000 x 1.03, leaving you with $4,120. As every year goes by, you can calculate what amount you can withdraw from your investment portfolio by taking the previous year's amount and adding inflation to it.

The specific technique has been around since the mid-nineties, and since it first became a popular guideline to ensure the safe spending of your retirement portfolio, it has been tested and challenged many times. Yet, it comes out on top every time as an effective way to ensure your retirement portfolio lasts up to as many as 30 years. Considering the general retirement age of 62, the 4% rule will ensure that you will have sufficient funds for the rest of your life.

Another benefit of this rule is that it can help you determine how much money you should save for retirement. It means that you have to calculate your expenses once you've retired. May I suggest that when you do this calculation, you prepare for the worst-case scenario rather than the best, then find the total of what it would cost you to live comfortably for a year in retirement? Now you have to work the sum backward to see how much you need for retirement so that 4% of this investment is enough to care for your financial needs. Let's say annually, your expenses total

$20,000. Then deduct any income you'll receive from sources outside your investment portfolio, like Social Security payments and pension funds. For our example, I will make this $10,000 per year, leaving you with $10,000 that you'll have to get from your investment portfolio. So, divide $10,000 by 0.04 to get to the total worth of your investment portfolio. In this case, an investment portfolio worth $250,000 will give you the lifestyle you desire during your golden years.

Let's Recap

It can be that finances have always been a matter of interest to you and that you are money savvy and know a lot about investments. However, many people have zero interest in investments and the stock market, and for them, it is much harder to make smart choices when it comes to retirement planning. Nonetheless, even if you are part of the latter group, you owe it to yourself and your loved ones to invest, first of all, your time to determine which option is the best for you and, secondly, funds to ensure you can live the life you desire once retired. Some of the options I've shared require a more hands-on approach, but you can also make proper provision for this time, even without being very involved in the process.

While financial planning for your retirement may be a complete pain for you, it is one of those areas in life where self-discipline and a smart approach pay off in many ways. So, free yourself of the stress caused by financial uncertainty and plan for financial freedom so that you can live longer and better.

6

TAKE CARE OF YOUR HOME ENVIRONMENT

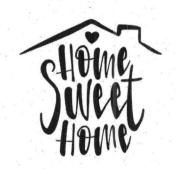

As you grow older, the condition in which you live will start to play a more important role in affecting your health and wellness. You will likely spend more time at home, and therefore it needs to be a place where you feel physically, mentally, and emotionally secure, but it should also be a place where you are happy and content to be. How do you feel about your home currently? Do you consider it a space where you merely come to sleep? Does it make you feel trapped or even vulnerable? Or, is your home your haven where you can rest and recuperate?

One of the main concerns older people face in their homes is the risk of falling. According to the CDC, there are annually 36 million incidents reported of older people falling. Of these incidents, 3 million were so severe that the patients ended up in emergency care, and 32,000 led to a fatality. The most significant risk of falling at an older age remains bone fractures, as one out of every five incidents caused bone fractures or head injuries (Keep on Your Feet—Preventing Older Adult Falls, 2020). Even if the safety in your home was not yet a matter of concern to you, these statistics serve as an eye-opener and are enough reason to cause anxiety and stress. So, let's see how you can increase safety in your home, one room at a time.

Room-by-Room Safety Guide

To ensure that you feel safe in every room of your home, you must consider the possible scenarios and even how those things that appear completely safe may cause a nasty fall.

Living Room

- The most important factors to consider in this specific space are the furniture, couches, and chairs, the quality of lighting you have in there, windows and the temperature control of the room, and then also the quality of floors and walkways, especially considering the kind of surface they have.
- Couches and chairs have to be of a height that is comfortable to sit down on and even more importantly,

to get up from. Older people often struggle to get up from seats that are very low or sunken in. Also, consider if there are armrests to help you push or pull yourself out of the seat. Ensure that all couches and chairs are stable seats and that they don't pose the risk of falling over. While heavy furniture pieces usually are much studier, they are hard to move around. Choose lightweight furniture that still offers that security.

- Lighting should provide clear visibility throughout the entire room. Therefore, take care that there are no dark spots in the room or even unwanted glare. It is best to have light switches in locations that are easy to reach, and where you don't have to walk through a dark room to get to the switch. Right at the door as you enter a room is the best place, but for people with mobility concerns, remote lighting may be the better alternative. Add additional lamps if needed and simply painting the room in a lighter shade, will also help to create a well-lit space.

- Windows and seals must provide a tight fit, preventing a draft that will cool the room down. When this is the case, you are likely to run up a high utility bill caused by heating expenses. To take this precaution up another notch, you can also install a door seal to prevent airflow from underneath the door. Keep your windows locked as a safety measure. Make sure that all heating devices are in a safe working state to prevent carbon poisoning. Curtains should not be too long as then they become trip hazards and don't place any objects in front of windows that will make it harder to reach your curtains.

- Floors and pathways should not have any obstructions that can cause a fall. This will mean you'll need to consider the risks any loose lying rugs may pose too. If you have hardwood floors in your home, always use non-slip wax on them, and try to avoid tiles or stone surfaces as these are cold and can be slippery. Install hand railings to offer additional support if you have trouble walking.

Bedrooms

- Of all the rooms in your home, this is the space where you really want to feel safe and secure. It should be a relaxing environment free from anything that might cause you anxiety or injury caused by a nasty fall. It is also a space where you may tend to store things for later use, but never do so, and eventually, it merely clutters up the space.
- Closets would be the first area to attend to. Get rid of clothes you are keeping for one day or anything else for that matter that doesn't have any sentimental value or purpose in your life. Make sure that your cupboards and storage spaces are packed in a manner that it is easy to get what you need.
- Lighting is another factor to consider here too. Ensure that you have enough lighting in your cupboard to be sure that you can find the things you are looking for easily. It is also best to have more than one light source in your room as at times you may need a lot of light to secure greater visibility and at times you just need low

light to create calming and peaceful surroundings. A lamp on your nightstand is so important, it should almost be a given. It allows you to just reach out your hand in the middle of the night and you'll have light to see. Nightlights will also help to prevent falls as you don't have to walk in your room in darkness.

- Floors in a bedroom are usually carpeted, any loose-lying carpets can pose a risk. So, rather keep these to the minimum. It is also best to keep the floor space clear of things like dirty laundry, shoes, or pillows.
- Bed heights are also a point to consider. It can be hard to get up from a lower bed. You can also consider having bed railings installed to make it easier to get up from your bed without losing your balance. When you look at your room, it should be a place without clutter, offering you a safe place to sleep and relax.

Bathrooms

- Bathrooms can easily be the space in your home posing the most risks for falling. These spaces are mostly tiled and can be slippery. Then there is also the risk of water spills that can make tiles even more slippery.
- Rubber mats on floors and in baths and shower floors reduce the risks of slipping and falling. They are relatively cheap to buy and easy to install.
- Railings in the bathroom, especially in the shower, next to baths, and even next to the toilet, will provide a secure place to hold onto or to help you get up if seated.

- Very low toilets can also pose the same challenges as a seat that is too low to get up from. In this case, hand railings would be essential.
- Taps should be clearly marked to indicate hot or cold.
- You can easily make your bathroom a safer place simply by setting your water thermostat to a maximum of 120°F, as this will prevent getting scalded.
- Showers are usually a safer alternative for older people, as bathtubs can be really hard to get up from, but you can overcome this challenge by installing secure seats in either your bath or shower. This will provide a safe space to sit down when you want to wash certain parts of your body and fear losing your balance when you would do so standing upright.
- If your medication cupboard is becoming cluttered, it is time to get rid of some items. Check the expiration date on all the containers and get rid of items that are no longer used. If your medicine cabinet is not big enough, it may be better to find a spot for them in the kitchen.
- Always keep your medication in its original packaging as this will make it easier to identify what it is. If your medication only has a prescription label on it, it may help to add another label that clearly states the name of the contents.
- Always keep medicine stored away where children and pets won't be able to reach it.

Kitchens

- If your storage space may be too high for you to reach, it poses a risk. Stretching to reach things high above your head may increase the risk of losing your balance and causing you to fall. Take care to install enough storage options in your kitchen that are within easy reach so that you don't have to get up onto a stool or a ladder.
- Try to get all work surfaces on a height that doesn't require standing bent over, or which will demand that you lift heavy items up high.
- Lazy Susans are a great way to provide access to all you need, and so are spice racks.
- Never keep your cleaning products near food items.
- Keep your refrigerator clean and prevent clutter by getting rid of old food as it expires. When you are storing leftover food, put them in airtight containers to prevent cross-contamination. Be sure to label these foods stating the contents and the date of storage.
- If you struggle to read labels, be sure to wear your reading glasses when cooking.

Fire Safety

- A house fire is a devastating event that should be avoided at all costs. Install working fire alarms in every room of your house, and fire extinguishers on each floor. Make sure that you know how to use these effectively. Fires can also be prevented by not having curtains near hot surfaces and avoiding burning candles as it is so easy to forget that you've lit them in the first place.

- Smoke and carbon monoxide alarms are a wonderful way to alert you and the fire department of fires as soon as they pose a risk. Get into the habit of checking and changing batteries in these devices at least twice a year.

- Consider having automatic shut-off valves installed on your stovetop and oven as this will automatically shut them off if you've forgotten about them, preventing them from being a risk.

Outside Your Home

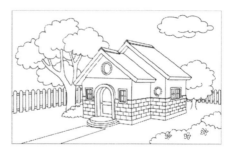

- The number of risk precautions you would need to consider drastically increase if you stay in an area where there is regular snowfall. Snow mats at all doors will help to prevent slips and falls, but you would also have to put other measures in place to avoid slipping outside on frozen surfaces and know how you'll clear the snow from your driveway or pathways.

- Other safety precautions would be to install a fence around your property to keep intruders out. Motion detectors linked to an alarm system will also give you peace of mind.
- Having motion detector lights around your home will also provide you with greater visibility to see if there are any threats outside of your home.
- Set your alarm system when you go to bed and always make sure that your system is connected to the necessary emergency response services. Older adults can also wear a panic button around their necks as help is only a simple press of a button away. This becomes even more vital to have if you plan to stay alone in your home.
- Doorbells that offer video footage can help you to determine who is at your door and if you choose to have one of the top-of-the-range options, you will be able to talk to the person too without opening your door and putting your life at risk. By having cameras installed around your home, you'll also be able to see who is outside and be able to call for help to protect you from any intruders.

Other Safety Tips

These tips include having the emergency contact numbers clearly listed in a place where it is easy to find. Many people prefer to have these posted on their fridges. You can also save these numbers on your phone. Also, make sure that you save them on a loved one's phone so that they know who to call if you are in distress. Another number you need to have clearly installed on your phone is your emergency contact person so that Emergency Response (ER) teams can quickly track down your loved ones.

If you have any allergies, it is best to wear a bracelet that will indicate to ER teams what they should be aware of if you are in no state to tell them yourself.

One great trick to ensure safe living and peace of mind for elderly people living on their own, is to have a contact chain. How it works is that older people have a communication list and every morning one person will contact the next. As soon as you've gotten your message that the person contacting you is fine, you reach out to another to indicate you are still fine and so the chain continues. If the chain is broken, then it is easy to track down who didn't respond and the agreement among group members is then to send emergency services to check on the person who broke the chain. Not knowing how long it will take anyone to check up on you to see if you are okay if something went wrong is a huge cause of concern for older people living on their own and simply being part of such a communication chain, can dissolve this stress.

Air Quality

We all assume that the air we breathe is relatively clean, right? This is even more so the case when we are at home. But what are we truly inhaling? What are the factors influencing the quality of air in your home? Air pollution is one of the most unnoticed types of pollution we expose ourselves to, for we simply can't see what we inhale, and often, air toxins don't have any odor either.

Asbestos

Did you know that asbestos is one of the leading causes of air pollution in your home? Asbestos is often used in building materials, flooring, and in fireproof solutions. As time passes, the asbestos fibers become loose and start floating in the air, where you of course inhale it. When you inhale these fibers, they get stuck in your lungs where they can cause scarring and inflammation, making them a major concern causing a range of health concerns like lung cancer. Therefore, it is vital to have your home regularly inspected for asbestos contamination and be sure that the air in your home is asbestos free.

Carbon Monoxide

The gas produced when burning fossil fuels like propane gas, oil, or gasoline is entirely odorless and you will not notice that there is a build-up of these gasses in your home. When you've suffered exposure to carbon monoxide, you are likely going to feel dizzy, have a headache, feel nauseous and eventually, it can be fatal. While exposure to carbon monoxide can be extremely dangerous, it is also quite easy to avoid. Refrain from burning any fuels where there is no proper ventilation. Even when you are using gas heaters or burners in your home, always make sure that there is a draft. If you can avoid using any of these in your home, rather do so and use them outside. Make sure you have carbon monoxide detectors in your home. Many insurance companies will require these.

Biological Pollutants

It is quite common to find spots of mold in homes across the globe and as this is such a common concern, we underestimate the risk it poses. Mold, bacteria, viruses, and allergens all fall under the category called biological pollutants. These all pose the threat of causing respiratory concerns, allergies, and even more serious health concerns. In homes, it is often the spores of mold that are the greatest matter of concern, as they float in the air and can even gather bacteria on their surface before we inhale them.

Excessive Moisture

Leaking water pipes or bathrooms with poor ventilation are some of the most common causes of excessive moisture in homes. Why is this such a high-risk concern? Surfaces with excessive moisture gather mold and dust. It provides a perfect breeding ground for mold to thrive while the dust becomes a place where dust mites will gather. When you inhale any of these, they can cause asthma and allergies. Prevent this from happening by repairing any leaks you notice. Increasing the airflow in these areas will help to dry them out or you can use a dehumidifier. When cooking and there is a lot of steam, it will help to open a window to create a draft, thus preventing condensation on your walls.

Volatile Organic Compounds

These usually evaporate from fluids or even solids like paint, pesticides, aerosol sprays, and even disinfectants. Use these in well-ventilated spaces. When exposed to these toxins, you will experience irritation of the mucus membranes in your nose, eyes, throat, and lungs.

Dust

If you live in an area where there is a lot of dust, or if you have pets, you are likely to have more dust gathered in your home. Carpets can be a concern as the dust gathers deep into the fibers and doesn't simply come out when vacuumed. This dust can cause allergies that make you more prone to develop respiratory concerns.

Pets

Pets create excessive dust, but they also shed their hair everywhere. Having pets would mean that you have to vacuum your carpets and furniture more often to prevent their fur from becoming airborne. Having air filters installed in your home and regularly replacing these filters will help to improve the quality of the air you breathe.

Radon

Radon is a chemical gas often found in basements or cellars. This gas is odorless, colorless, and tasteless, making it very hard to detect without professional equipment. However, radon is a radioactive gas that causes lung cancer, so have your home regularly checked by a professional to be sure you don't expose yourself or your loved ones to this high-risk gas.

Poor Ventilation

It is tempting to keep all doors and windows closed, especially if it is cold, but a home with poor ventilation is a place where you will have more dust gathering and bad gasses as well as moisture building up. These are all just concerns threatening your overall health and wellness. While it is always good to give your home a bit of a draft whenever possible, you can also choose to install a ventilation system that will keep the quality of your air healthy to breathe.

How to Determine the Quality of Air in Your Home

How would you know if the air quality in your home needs attention? In most cases, you will start to experience symptoms you are not used to. For example, if you suddenly start to struggle with coughing, sneezing, or asthma symptoms without any reason, it may be due to some form of air pollution in your home. Other more severe symptoms include feeling dizzy, nauseous, or irritation in your eyes, throat, and nose.

If the above is the case, cut down on the use of pollutants in your home. It is also a good time to call in a professional to check the quality of your air and they'll be able to identify the source of your concern. Until then, ensure there is enough ventilation, see if you can determine where these pollutants escape from, or if your concern is linked to excessive moisture, get a dehumidifier to dry the air in the meantime. Another beautiful accessory that does wonders for the quality of the air you breathe in your home, is indoor plants. So, add some plants to your indoor spaces to help keep your air clean.

Water Safety

While most homes in the Western world have access to fresh water to drink, there are sometimes factors that can affect the quality of your water even when you are thinking that it is perfectly fine to have. It can happen at times when water supply sources get polluted, or when the structure of the pipes bringing water to your home is compromised. However, it is not only polluted drinking water that can be a cause of concern, as any mass of water collected in your home, can become the breeding ground for microorganisms that can cause a range of health concerns. Yet, here too, there are several steps you can take to ensure your home is a risk-free place where you have easy access to clean water and no stagnant water turns into a high-risk zone.

Invest in Test Kits

There are several kits available on the market which will give you an instant indication of the quality of your water. They are affordable and easy to use. If you find that there is a problem with your water, apply the following preventative steps to keep your water safe and your health protected until a professional can come and investigate your property to determine the cause of concern.

Boil Your Drinking Water

Even though it can be time-consuming to boil and cool down all your drinking water, it is a sure and simple way to ensure that your water is safe. When boiling water, you are killing all possible germs and bacteria that may have contaminated it. Make sure that your water boils for at least a minute before allowing it to cool down. When you are letting this water cool, make sure it is covered so that no dust can gather on the surface and prevent future contamination.

Filter Your Water

While boiling may remove any threats posed by living organisms, it doesn't remove other contaminants like dust or sediment. Therefore, filter your water before boiling it to be completely sure that it is safe to drink. You can use a piece of clean cloth to filter it, but you can also have water filters installed on your taps. These filters need to be cleaned regularly, otherwise, they won't be of any aid, but when they are clean, they offer you the certainty of having safe drinking water.

Water Aerators

By installing water aerators onto your taps, you increase the amount of air that is in the water making it a safer option to drink. These nifty devices simply break up air and fuse it with your water. The greatest benefit you'll enjoy from such an installation is that it removes the risks and the taste of chlorine in the water. Chlorine is an essential component to keep drinking water clean and safe, but it can also create several other health concerns if not managed effectively. By having aerators installed in your home, you are taking control of your water management in this regard.

Clean Faucets Regularly

The calcium in water can cause a build-up in your faucets that can become a concern for contamination. Therefore, if you are unsure about how to do it yourself, get a plumber to service your taps regularly to give you peace of mind. However, faucets make up only one part of the system bringing water to your home and many other parts of this system can be deteriorating too. For a couple of years already, there has been a growing concern regarding lead and copper exposure in old and worn pipes. A large part of water distribution systems across the entire nation consists of copper pipes and if you are concerned about the quality of the water you get in your home, it is best to have it tested or to report your concerns at your local water provider. You can also check to see if you rely on any copper pipes on your property to carry drinking water. Copper pipes tend to get a blue-green tone when they are getting old. If you do notice such pipes, it is best to get a professional to replace these pipes for you with a safer solution.

Water Heaters

It is not only the water that you drink that poses a threat to your health and safety. No, you also need to consider the water that is standing in containers that may cause pollution. For example, water heaters have to have the water in them replaced regularly. If not, the water can become infected with germs and bacteria and when heated, your air will be polluted too.

Ponds and Outside Dams

Outside ponds or dams can be another place where bacteria can gather. Therefore, it is best to clean these spaces regularly too. They are exposed to dirt and natural organisms that can pose a threat to your health. Stagnant ponds are a prime breeding ground for mosquitoes.

Keep Storm Water Drains Clean

It can be so easy to neglect these drains on your property for few people ever consider the fact that your stormwater drains can impact the quality of your drinking water. If these aren't clean, they can contribute to groundwater pollution. It often happens that the contaminants from your house water sewerage end up in these drains and from here can easily be spread to aquatic ecosystems. While it may initially not seem as if a little contamination of household cleaning products can do any harm, these toxins gradually build up in the environment and pose a major concern, threatening the security of clean drinking water in the future.

Septic Tank Maintenance

Septic tanks can also create a high-risk situation threatening the state of groundwater. These tanks tend to form a build-up that can clog the leach field if not cleared out. When this happens, you'll have little control over where water from your septic tank leaks into. While this can create a major health risk in your back garden, it is also a threat that has lasting consequences. The best approach is to use the correct additives that support the break-up taking place in these tanks and to have your tank checked regularly by a professional. If you have any concerns in this regard, it is best to call in an expert.

Water Softener

Do you stay in an area with water that is naturally high in minerals? These minerals tend to gather in pipes and taps where it forms a layer of crystals, impacting the quality of your water. This is when a water softener can come in handy to improve the quality of your drinking water. The water softener removes most minerals like magnesium, calcium, and even iron, making your water taste better and it protects your taps, pipes, and equipment from damage.

Let's Recap

When it comes to ensuring that your home is a safe and friendly environment to stay in, it may initially appear as if all is in good order. However, the message that I wanted to bring across in this chapter is that often, we may assume that matters are just fine, but they are not. While you can call in an expert to take care of any of the concerns I've highlighted in this text, most of these you'll be able to take care of yourself. Through simple maintenance and greater awareness of your surroundings, your home can be a safe place to be, offering you protection from a range of risks.

CONCLUSION

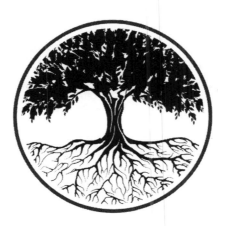

We make an endless number of choices daily throughout our lives. Yet, most of the time, we don't consider the impact these choices have on our lives simply because we assume that most of them don't affect us. It is often the case that only later in life when we start to notice how the impact of our choices has been building up to create a specific situation. Then we begin to wonder if it was the best choice to make back then or even regret some of these choices.

When we grow older, it is easy to get entangled in stress and anxiety, for we realize that time is limited and life doesn't include any retakes. We can't just step back in time and choose to do better when we are old enough to know better. Coupled with this type of stress is that you may not know what you will do with the rest of your life or even believe there is nothing left for you to do, that being older means living an empty life without purpose.

If this is the position you found yourself in when you started to read this book, I hope my words, tips, and guidance can convince you of two things.

First, I wanted you to realize that it is never too late to change the outcome. It doesn't matter how long you've waited to consider what you need to do to make your golden years brilliant. It is never too late. There will always be a day when you look back on today and may wish that you made smarter choices *back then*. So, let today count and make informed decisions about your future.

The second point I wanted to bring up is that many of the fears you may link to growing older are based on your perception of this stage in life. These are often uninformed perceptions. It is a state fueled by a lack of knowledge. So, regardless of whether the topic was physical or mental health, being socially connected, or securing financial stability, it was all done based on sharing what you should be aware of and how to address the challenges you may notice.

As we grow older, we become wiser too. Through this wisdom, we learn how to distinguish between the things we can control and to take steps to manage them to the best of our ability, but also to determine what we can't control and to accept them as part of life. Therefore, every word in this book was written from the perspective that we may not have any control over aging. We are all growing older daily, but instead of dreading getting old, we can see it as a blessing to have a long life. We can extend our life expectancy and make the time we have as older people a rewarding and fulfilling stage in life. You have complete control over your current lifestyle, the choices you make regarding your finances, how well you plan, and how you take care of your home. Transform your choices and habits now so that they contribute to your life instead of chiseling years off your life expectancy. And always remember that even if your choices seem like they have little to no impact on your life today, the effect compounds over time, and the benefit you are working for today, becomes yours to reap in your future.

I want to conclude with the following words of wisdom from Ralph Waldo Emerson, "Getting old is a fascinating thing. The older you get, the older you want to get."

If you feel inspired and ready to embrace growing older in the best possible way after reading this book, please leave a positive review on *Amazon* and help me spread the word that through proper planning, you can remove the sting of aging and turn old age into the best time of your life.

PLEASE LEAVE A REVIEW

If you have found this book to be of value so far, please take a moment right now and leave an honest review of this book

This will take you less than a minute of your time. All you have to do is to leave a review.

Please go to the page on Amazon (or where you purchased this book) and leave a review.

Alternatively, you can scan the QR code below to land on the review page:

Thank you for your kindness.

ABOUT THE AUTHOR

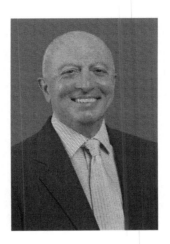

Dr. Naghshineh, a retired chair and professor of Mechanical Engineering, has been a health and fitness enthusiast for most of his life. When not writing or conducting research at the university, you can find him and his wife exercising, playing tennis, or enjoying time spent with friends and family.

The author specializes in books about diet and wellness, aging, and exercise routines for seniors. Since his retirement from academia, he has turned his skills in academic research to improving his own health and the health of those around him. This book is the culmination of his research into aging and how one can live longer as a healthy individual.

BIBLIOGRAPHY

Active social life may help you live longer. (2019). Harvard T. H. Chan. https://www.hsph.harvard.edu/news/hsph-in-the-news/active-social-life-longevity/#

Anderson, G. (2022, July 7). *5 Reasons older adults should aim to live longer.* Home Care Assistance. https://www.homecareassistancehuntsville.com/why-seniors-should-live-longer/

Barron, J. (2020, February 16). *How your mindset might affect your longevity, vitality and your mood!!* Dr Jill Baron. https://drjillbaron.com/how-your-mindset-might-affect-your-longevity-vitality-and-your-mood/

Beckman, K. (2016, May 27). *9 Factors that affect longevity.* ThinkAdvisor. https://www.thinkadvisor.com/2016/05/27/9-factors-that-affect-longevity/

Bemis, E. (2019, March 5). *6 Best cognitive games and activities for seniors.* UMH. https://www.umh.org/assisted-independent-living-blog/6-best-cognitive-games-and-activities-for-seniors#

Berger, R. (2022, August 18). *What is the 4% rule for retirement withdrawals?* Forbes Advisor. https://www.forbes.com/advisor/retirement/four-percent-rule-retirement/

Best, T. (2020, December 3). *Your mindset is the single biggest weapon you have – use it wisely.* Association of MBAs. https://www.associationofmbas.com/your-mindset-is-the-single-biggest-weapon-you-have-use-it-wisely/

Better health channel. (n.d.). *Strong relationships, strong health.* Better Health Channel. https://www.betterhealth.vic.gov.au/health/HealthyLiving/Strong-relationships-strong-health

Cognitive Stimulation Therapy. (n.d.). Psychologytoday. https://www.psychologytoday.com/us/therapy-types/cognitive-stimulation-therapy#how-its-used

Contributors, W. E. (2021). *What to Know About Cognitive Decline in Older Adults.* WebMD. https://www.webmd.com/healthy-aging/what-to-know-about-cognitive-decline-in-older-adults

Countries with the lowest life expectancy worldwide 2022. (n.d.). Statista. https://www.statista.com/statistics/274521/countries-with-the-lowest-life-expectancy-worldwide/#:~:text=Males%20born%20in%20the%20Lesotho

Crider, D. (2021, April 7). 26 Motivational running quotes to inspire your best. *Running Glow.* https://www.runningglow.com/26-motivational-running-quotes/

Dong, T. (2022, September 20). *7 High-return, low-risk investments for retirees.* US News.

https://money.usnews.com/investing/investing-advice/articles/high-return-low-risk-investments-for-retirees

Drinko, C. (n.d.). *What is a fixed mindset and can you change it?* Lifehack. https://www.lifehack.org/871367/fixed-mindset#how-can-you-change-a-fixed-mindset

The 15 places where people live the longest. (n.d.). HGTV. https://www.hgtv.com/lifestyle/health-and-wellness/places-where-people-live-the-longest-pictures

Five Brain stimulating activities for older adults. (n.d.). Careasone. https://careasone.com/blog/5-brain-stimulating-activities-for-older-adults/

Five Factors that affect indoor air quality at home. (2020, February 29). Extreme Air & Electric, Inc. https://www.extremeairandelectric.com/article/5-factors-that-affect-indoor-air-quality-at-home

Fonville, M. (2020, February 2). *9 Reasons why retirement planning is important.* Covenant. https://www.covenantwealthadvisors.com/post/9-reasons-why-retirement-planning-is-important

Four Main causes of indoor air pollutants and easy ways to address them. (2022, December 14). Hepacart. https://www.hepacart.com/blog/4-main-causes-of-indoor-air-pollutants-and-easy-ways-to-address-them

Fuhrman, J. (n.d.). *The 10 best foods for longevity.* Strong Body and Mind. https://www.denverhealthmedicalplan.org/blog/10-best-foods-longevity

Gunnars, K. (2021, May 13). *10 Evidence-based health benefits of intermittent fasting.* Healthline. https://www.healthline.com/nutrition/10-health-benefits-of-intermittent-fasting#TOC_TITLE_HDR_2

Hartman, R. (2021a, January 6). *20 Steps to take when preparing for retirement.* US News & World Report. https://money.usnews.com/money/retirement/401ks/articles/steps-to-take-when-preparing-for-retirement

Hartman, R. (2021b, March 17). *How to create a retirement budget.* US News & World Report. https://money.usnews.com/money/retirement/baby-boomers/articles/how-to-create-a-retirement-budget

How much physical activity do older adults need? (2022, June 3). Centers for Disease Control and Prevention. https://www.cdc.gov/physicalactivity/basics/older_adults/index.htm#

How the aging brain affects thinking. (n.d.). National Institute on Aging. https://www.nia.nih.gov/health/how-aging-brain-affects-thinking#

How to overcome your self-limiting beliefs around age. (2019, May 1). So Chickie. https://www.sochickie.com/anti-aging/how-to-overcome-your-self-limiting-beliefs-around-age/

Hull, M. (2022, April 28). *Poor mental health's devastating impacts on life expectancy.* The Recovery Village. https://www.therecoveryvillage.com/mental-health/mental-health-impact-on-life-expectancy/

Jones, R. (n.d.). *9 easy tips on how to improve water quality in your home.* Phyxter Home Services. https://phyxter.ai/blog/improve-the-quality-of-your-water

Kagan, J. (2022, December 16). *5 Key retirement-planning steps to take.* Investopedia. https://www.investopedia.com/articles/retirement/11/5-steps-to-retirement-plan.asp

Keep on your feet—preventing older adult falls. (2020, December 6). Centers for Disease and Control Prevention. https://www.cdc.gov/injury/features/older-adult-falls/index.html#

Key, J. (n.d.). *16 Benefits of exercise for the elderly.* The Care Workers Charity. https://www.thecareworkerscharity.org.uk/blog/benefits-of-exercise-for-the-elderly/

Klodas, E. (2015, May 8). *The 4 pillars of healthy longevity.* Step One Foods. https://www.steponefoods.com/blogs/news/the-4-pillars-of-healthy-longevity

Klodas, E. (2020, September 9). *These 4 pillars of longevity support the fountain of youth.* Sixty and Me. https://sixtyandme.com/these-4-pillars-of-longevity-support-the-fountain-of-youth/

Lamb-Balfour, T. (2022, October 5). *Retirement investments: A beginner's guide.* Nerd-Wallet. https://www.nerdwallet.com/article/investing/retirement-investments-beginners-guide

Lifestyle medicine pillars. (n.d.). Lifestyle Medicine. https://longevity.stanford.edu/life-style-medicine-2/lifestyle-pillars/#

Longevity - an Overview | ScienceDirect Topics. (n.d.). Science Direct. https://www.sci-encedirect.com/topics/agricultural-and-biological-sciences/longevity

Mapes, J. (2020, January 28). *11 Strategies to establish social connections for your life.* The Good Men Project. https://goodmenproject.com/guy-talk/11-strategies-to-establish-social-connections-for-your-life-fiff/

Meyer, S. (2022, September 21). *Comprehensive room-by-room home safety guide for older adults.* The Zebra. https://www.thezebra.com/resources/home/senior-home-safety-guide/

Mind. (2022, March). *Signs and symptoms of stress.* Mind. https://www.mind.org.uk/information-support/types-of-mental-health-problems/stress/signs-and-symptoms-of-stress/

Mindset. (n.d.). Cale Learning Enhancement. https://inside.ewu.edu/calelearning/psychological-skills/mindset/

Mr Rooter. (2020, July 28). *How to improve water quality in 5 easy steps.* Mr. Rooter Plumbing. https://www.mrrooter.com/about/blog/2020/july/how-to-improve-water-quality-in-5-easy-steps/

Naghshineh, K. (2022a). *Never Fear Falling Again.* Self-published. https://www.amazon.com/dp/B0B1N32HDZ

Naghshineh, K. (2022b). *Intermittent Fasting: Beginner's Guide to Weight Loss for Men and Women Over 50*. Self-published. https://www.amazon.com/dp/B0BNQGY936

Nunez, K. (2020, September 10). *The benefits of guided imagery and how to do it*. Healthline. https://www.healthline.com/health/guided-imagery

Orem, T. (2023, January 5). *5 steps to retirement planning in 2023*. NerdWallet. https://www.nerdwallet.com/article/investing/retirement-planning-an-introduction

Perkins, K. (2022, January 4). *Chronic stress can reduce lifespan, says recent Yale study*. Connecticut Public. https://www.ctpublic.org/news/2022-01-04/chronic-stress-can-reduce-lifespan-says-recent-yale-study

Ralph Waldo Emerson quote: "Getting old is a fascination thing. The older you get, the older you want to get." (n.d.). Quotefancy. https://quotefancy.com/quote/893314/Ralph-Waldo-Emerson-Getting-old-is-a-fascination-thing-The-older-you-get-the-older-you#

Ramsey Solutions. (2022, September 30). *How to create a retirement budget*. Ramsey. https://www.ramseysolutions.com/retirement/how-much-money-will-you-need-in-retirement

Royal, J. (2023, January 1). *9 Best retirement plans in 2023*. Bankrate. https://www.bankrate.com/retirement/best-retirement-plans/

Saweetie Quotes. (n.d.). BrainyQuote. https://www.brainyquote.com/quotes/saweetie_1038593?src=t_longevity

Scott, E. (2022, October 19). *18 Effective stress relief strategies*. Verywell Mind. https://www.verywellmind.com/tips-to-reduce-stress-3145195

Seegert, L. (2021, June 1). *4 Ways exercise helps fight aging*. Time. https://time.com/6053055/how-exercise-fights-aging/

Segal, J. (2022, December 5). *Stress symptoms, signs, and causes*. Helpguide. https://www.helpguide.org/articles/stress/stress-symptoms-signs-and-causes.htm

Segal, T. (2023, January 8). *6 Surprising facts about retirement*. Investopedia. https://www.investopedia.com/articles/retirement/110116/6-surprising-facts-about-retirement.asp

Selig, M. (2022, September 30). *9 Longevity habits for a happy and healthy older age*. Psychology Today. https://www.psychologytoday.com/us/blog/changepower/202209/9-longevity-habits-happy-and-healthy-older-age

Shaw, R. (2022, December 8). *Paying off debt in retirement*. InCharge Debt Solutions. https://www.incharge.org/debt-relief/paying-debt-after-retirement/

Shrikant, A. (2022, August 29). *The "U-shaped happiness curve" theory says your 40s will be your unhappiest age—here's why that's wrong, according to a therapist*. CNBC. https://www.cnbc.com/2022/08/29/u-shaped-happiness-curve-why-your-40s-will-actually-be-satisfying.html

Stanley, A. (2018, February 1). *21 Best ways to meet new friends in a new city or town*.

MAS Medical Staffing. https://www.masmedicalstaffing.com/blog/best-ways-to-meet-new-friends-in-a-new-city/

Suknanan, J. (2022, November 30). *What is the 4% rule and how can it help you save for retirement?* CNBC. https://www.cnbc.com/select/what-is-the-4-percent-retirement-savings-rule/

Sutton, J. (2018, February 23). *10 techniques to manage stress & 13 quick tips.* Positive Psychology. https://positivepsychology.com/stress-management-techniques-tips-burn-out/

Tennessee, S. C. of M. (n.d.). *The Sleep Habits That May Help, or Hurt, Longevity | Sleep Centers of Middle Tennessee.* Sleepcenterinfo.com. https://sleepcenterinfo.com/blog/the-sleep-habits-that-may-help-or-hurt-longevity/#

32 room-by-room home safety tips. (2015, August 29). The Caregiver Space. https://www.thecaregiverspace.org/32-room-by-room-home-safety-tips/

Tuttle, C. (2021, March 8). *Top 5 limiting beliefs that age you.* Carol Tuttle. https://ct.liveyourtruth.com/top-5-limiting-beliefs-that-age-you/

Watters, A. (2017, July 21). *8 Easy ways to improve your water quality.* Scadata. https://scadata.net/easy-ways-improve-water-quality/

What are the 4 major indoor air pollutants. (2020, September 18). Savannah Air Factory. https://savannahairfactory.com/what-are-the-4-major-indoor-air-pollutants/

What is cognitive stimulation? (n.d.). HappyNeuron Pro. https://www.happyneuronpro.com/en/info/cognitive-stimulation/

Williams, C. (2022, August 27). *6 Ways the Mediterranean diet helps you live longer, according to a dietitian.* EatingWell. https://www.eatingwell.com/article/7996072/ways-the-mediterranean-diet-helps-you-live-longer-according-to-a-dietitian/

Worldometer. (2020). *Life expectancy of the world population.* Worldometers. https://www.worldometers.info/demographics/life-expectancy/

Zhavoronkov, A. (n.d.). *Don't let the old man in: How to develop a longevity mindset and fight psychological aging?* Forbes. https://www.forbes.com/sites/alexzhavoronkov/2022/02/07/dont-let-the-old-man-in-how-to-develop-a-longevity-mindset-and-fight-psychological-aging/